SPEECHLESS DREAM

NARRATIVES ON AUTISM,
INCLUSION AND HOPE

CHANDRA LEBENHAGEN | ANANTHA KRISHNAMURTHY | JANANI RAMANATH | ROBERT CHOATE

◆ FriesenPress

One Printers Way
Altona, MB R0G 0B0
Canada

www.friesenpress.com

Copyright © 2022 by Chandra Lebenhagen, Anantha Krishnamurthy, Janani Ramanath and Robert Choate

First Edition — 2022

All rights reserved.

No part of this publication may be reproduced in any form, or by any means, electronic or mechanical, including photocopying, recording, or any information browsing, storage, or retrieval system, without permission in writing from FriesenPress.

ISBN
978-1-03-915405-6 (Hardcover)
978-1-03-915404-9 (Paperback)
978-1-03-915406-3 (eBook)

1. MEDICAL, CAREGIVING

Distributed to the trade by The Ingram Book Company

SPEECHLESS DREAM

NARRATIVES ON AUTISM,
INCLUSION AND HOPE

CHANDRA LEBENHAGEN | ANANTHA KRISHNAMURTHY | JANANI RAMANATH | ROBERT CHOATE

Table of Contents

Foreword	vii
Author's Note	xi
Four People, Four Stories	1
The Beginning of Our Story	3
Chapter 1: Chinook	11
Chapter 2: Elevators	29
Chapter 3: Conversion	51
Chapter 4: Holes	75
Chapter 5: Light	95
Chapter 6: Manual	117
Chapter 7: Final Reflections	133
References	147
About the Authors	159

FOREWORD

I'm a developmental psychologist. Questions about how culture and context shape who we are, and about how we shape culture and context loom large in my research. Over the course of my career, I have had the opportunity to get to know many nonspeaking autistic people and their families—as friends, neighbors, self-advocates, students in a seminar on autism I teach at the University of Virginia, and as collaborators in research in my lab. They are the inspiration for the work I do.

The variability in autism is real. But in all my interactions with nonspeaking folks, there is a clear through-line: They have an intense desire to be included, to be given the same opportunities as everyone else, and to be accepted. Who wouldn't want these things?

Unfortunately, historically and for the most part even today, authentic inclusion and acceptance of autistic people are rare. Instead and unrealistically, autistic people are expected to change, to conform to non-autistic ways of being, to somehow demonstrate that they are "ready" to be included. You don't have to be a psychologist to see how these kinds of messages, received day in and day out, in ways implicit and explicit, would wear a person down.

The good news is that things don't have to be this way. Culture and context shape who we are, but we can choose to shape culture and context in progressive ways. We can choose to create authentically welcoming and inclusive schools and communities, places, and spaces where people are accepted for who they are and provided the support they need to thrive.

The book you are about to read is a beautiful account of four individuals' intersecting journeys as they work together to create such places and spaces, particularly in a school setting. The protagonist is Anantha, a remarkable nonspeaking autistic young man, whose patience, and determination know no bounds as he encounters and overcomes roadblock after roadblock on his journey to be taken seriously. In this account, he is joined on his journey by three allies: his mother (Janani) and two inclusion specialists (Robert and Chandra).

Together, these four authors weave a narrative that is, at once, heartbreaking and hopeful. It is heartbreaking because the exclusion, othering, and presumption of incompetence that Anantha describes having experienced is something that no child (or adult) should ever be subjected to. But it is also hopeful because it provides an example of how different things can be when erroneous assumptions about nonspeaking autistic people are put aside, when access to an effective means of communication is provided, and (at the risk of being cliché) when people work together to support each other.

Foreword

Early in the book, Anantha describes himself as "the boy without a user manual." And toward the end, he provides that manual. It has just three instructions: 1. Accept me, 2. Presume I'm competent, and 3. Show me love and kindness. Isn't that the manual for all of us?

Vikram K. Jaswal, Ph.D.
Professor of Psychology
University of Virginia

AUTHOR'S NOTE

As an educator, I have worked alongside autistic children, youth, adults, and their families for over 20 years. I have also researched the inclusive education experiences of autistic youth in Canada. Hence, I am keenly aware of the disconnect between theories and practices of inclusive education and the experiences of autistic students.

I proposed writing this book together because, over one school year, I observed critical shifts in educator views on belonging, equity, and inclusion in the life of a minimally speaking autistic boy named Anantha. Over time, these small shifts amounted to sizeable improvements in Anantha's academic achievements, sense of school belonging, and quality of relationships with teachers and peers. The benefits of our unique and uncomplicated approach extended beyond Anantha's successes to visible changes in teacher attitudes on communication, regulation, behaviour, dignity, friendships, learning, assessment— and what it means to be included from the perspective of a semi-speaking autistic boy.

Sharing our journey through stories is our way to commemorate our successes, challenge discourse on normative ability, and create provocations for researchers, jurisdictional leaders, and educators to re-examine their beliefs so that more students with disabilities feel a greater sense of acceptance, belonging, and inclusion in school.

Chandra Lebenhagen, EdD

FOUR PEOPLE, FOUR STORIES

THE BEGINNING OF OUR STORY

This book weaves the narratives of four people —Anantha, his mother Janani[1], Robert, and me. Our lives intersected in the autumn of 2020 because Anantha, a minimally speaking autistic boy, was about to attend a science program for his grade seven year. Anantha is intelligent, wise, compassionate, creative, playful, and deeply expressive. However, like many students who don't fit the mould, Anantha, and his parents, have spent countless hours and immense energy pushing back against ableist systems and practices that perpetuate difference as deficit-type thinking.

Ableism is a form of discrimination that devalues persons with disabilities resulting in practices that aim to remediate or cure a person's disability (Hehir, 2002) and is reflected in medical, social, and education systems that implicitly and explicitly limit the authentic participation of disabled people (MTOWN97, 2019). For example, ableism is represented in educators' beliefs that

---

1 Anantha's father, Diwakar, also shared his ideas, experiences, and perspectives at each stage in the book's development and was Anantha's main communication partner.

the barrier to inclusion "resides within the student and that the *student* must overcome those barriers" (Graham et al., 2020, p. 28) to be successfully included in school. Robert, Anantha's in-school champion, has been pivotal in helping Anantha's school team reframe views of disability and autonomy so that Anantha attends school in meaningful and dignified ways.

While this book focuses on the narratives of four people, we would like to acknowledge that many others have been vital supporters of Anantha's success at home and school, including speech-language therapists, occupational therapists, psychologists, teachers, and school leaders.

THE WAY WE CAME TOGETHER

To guide the weaving together of our stories, we needed to find a process that created a safe space for us to share ideas and feedback while at the same time offering both structure and flow. Anantha was the first to write entries and created a title for each chapter, which provided the overall framework for this book. Every two to three weeks, Janani, Robert, and I wrote a piece inspired by Anantha's writing. The group would send me their draft at the end of the writing period. I would compile individual narratives into one-chapter, complete minor edits, and re-send an updated draft to the group to review before our next virtual meeting. We repeated this pattern for a little over one year. Our method of co-authorship was organic, and we agreed that minimal content editing would occur as we wanted each of our stories and the way we told them to remain authentic as possible.

Each chapter begins with a poem written by Anantha and continues in a journal-like format, where Anantha, Janani, and Robert share personal reflections and experiences. I conclude each chapter by occasionally sharing a personal experience; however, I mainly connect themes discussed by Anantha, Janani, and Robert with current research. You will find Anantha's and Janani's stories follow a birth to a present-day timeline, and Robert and my stories begin when we were introduced to Anantha, which was September 2020, his grade seven-year.

THE LEGITIMACY OF AUTISTIC VOICE

Toward the end of our second meeting, Janani raised a question about the legitimacy of Anantha's voice and, therefore, his story because Anantha uses different communication techniques, including a letter board, a laptop, and Augmentative and Alternative Communication (AAC) software on his iPad. I wasn't surprised by Janani's question because I was familiar with several other autistic people sharing experiences where the legitimacy of their messages was doubted because the messages were not spoken, or physical support was received to type.

The controversy specifically relates to methods of facilitated communication using a letter board. Individuals receive motor support to point at letters through gentle arm and hand touches (ISAAC, 2014; Mitchell, 2017). Some people defend that the communication partner, not the communicator, creates messages either partially or whole (Ganz, 2014; Saloviita et al., 2014).

Adding to outsider suspicion is when an autistic person interchangeably uses speaking and non-speaking modes of communication. Those who speak to communicate might question why an autistic person can speak some days or in some situations but not others—often assuming that this inconsistency is due to choice, manipulation or even bad behaviour on the part of the autistic person.

Independent verbal communication is society's expected and preferred mode and is founded on ableist constructs of "normal" intellect, eye gaze, motor planning, and rules on reciprocity and time. Using head-mounted eye tracking technology, researchers have challenged questions about the communicative agency of non and minimally speaking autistics, finding that in response to novel questions, participants looked at a letter approximately half a second before pointing to it and rarely made spelling mistakes (Jaswal et al., 2020). Therefore, based on measures of accuracy, timing, and patterns of visual fixation, research has confirmed that autistic people who receive support via communication partners are, in fact, independently producing their messages.

Preference for spoken communication is reflected in schools and classrooms, meaning oral speech is a privileged representation of intellect and reasoning ability (Bergenmar et al., 2015; St. Pierre, 2015; Tisdall, 2012). Autistic teen Ido Kedar (2018) offers a personal message to those who seek to understand autism and communication from an insider perspective:

> *There is an overwhelming need for professionals to learn about autism from those who live it and can describe it in words. I am referring to the non-speaking typer who tries to explain autism from the inside out. There are now quite a few of us, and the number is growing. Our messages are always the same. Intact mind/disobeying body. Smart head/dumb body. Thinking mind/non-thinking motor system. Not speaking is not the same as not thinking (para. 2).*

While the legitimacy of non and minimally speaking voice continues to be debated amongst researchers, educators, clinicians, parents, and speaking and non-speaking autistics, we must not forget that communication is a human right. Article 13 of *The Convention on the Rights of the Child* (1989) states:

> *"The child shall have the right to freedom of expression; this shall include the freedom to seek, receive and impart information and ideas of all kinds, regardless of frontiers, either orally, in writing or in print, in the form of art, or through any other media of the child's choice."*

Hence, my reply to Janani was unconcerned with the communication skeptic. Like many historical stances that question the ability and legitimacy of the disabled mind and body, ideas surrounding the legitimacy of non and minimally speaking voice will continue to shift as insider perspectives outweigh outsider assumptions and biases.

AUTISTIC PERSON OR PERSON WITH AUTISM?

There is also debate on the use of identity-first or person-first language in the autism community. Researchers have explored the viewpoints of autistic people, parents, and professionals to better understand the reasons underlying their preferences. Findings show that most autistic people prefer identity-first language, and parents and professionals prefer to use person-first language (Kenny et al., 2015). Parents defend that the person should come first, not their diagnosis and reason that "the person with autism is a person-first and their condition second" (Kenny et al., 2015, p.9). Lydia Brown, autistic author and advocate shares her perspective on how language shapes her autistic identity:

> ...when we say "Autistic person," we recognize, affirm, and validate an individual's identity as an Autistic person. We recognize the value and worth of that individual as an Autistic person — that being Autistic is not a condition absolutely irreconcilable with regarding people as inherently valuable and worth something. We affirm the individual's potential to grow and mature, to overcome challenges and disability, and to live a meaningful life as an Autistic. Ultimately, we are accepting that the individual is different

> *from non-Autistic people—and that that's not a tragedy, and we are showing that we are not afraid or ashamed to recognize that difference (Brown, 2011, para. 18).*

While discussions on the use of identity-first versus person-first language continue, we must consider how language conveys our beliefs on disability, acceptance, and belonging and how this ultimately affects the identity of autistic people. Thus, aligning with Anantha's preference for identity-first language, terms such as Autism Spectrum Disorder (ASD) or person with autism are avoided throughout these pages unless specifically used to support the main idea, such as the concept of ableism.

THE SUBJECTIVITY OF STORIES

Meaning-making is always context-bound and influenced by time, space, people, and politics. Personal accounts are, therefore, "open-ended, inconclusive and ambiguous, subject to multiple interpretations" (Denzin, 1981, p. 81). Our interpretations and retelling of our stories are not free from bias and are influenced by our histories and beliefs. In the research world, hermeneutics is a method used to dissect our roles within an experience to question rules and norms that guide our actions and our beliefs, attitudes, values, and assumptions (French & Hankins, 2003). In the teaching world, this process is called critical reflection. Through various methods, teachers are challenged to reflect on their biases and assumptions and consider how this impacts the pedagogical practices used in the classroom (Brookfield, 2017).

We believe stories are powerful agents of change; they help us disentangle biases and reshape our belief systems through unfamiliar, sometimes inconvenient truths. Whether you are a researcher, administrator, teacher, parent, or student, we hope our stories create provocations for you to (re)consider your beliefs and assumptions about autistic people and perceptions of ability. We also hope that our stories inspire you to find ways to make space for the authentic inclusion of autistic people that respects their identity, dignity, and voice.

CHAPTER 1: CHINOOK

Lullaby
(to a newborn autistic baby)

Welcome sweet angel.
As time flies, so will you.
Clip your wings,
I shall not.
Capable you are
Of deeds most heavenly.
Devil's apostles may
Darken your sky.
Clouding you with
Labels aplenty.
Fear not,
For they do that
To feel safe in their dim dungeons.
Sleep safe knowing that
I will be a candle
To light up your soul
'Til my last radiant flicker.

~Anantha

Anantha

MY ARRIVAL IN 2007

The Chinook arch spread across Calgary's sky as if to welcome my arrival. Chinooks are God's gift of warmth for Calgary, bestowing regular relief to a city reeling from a seemingly endless winter. My birth too appeared as a gift to my parents. "What a blessed child!" they exalted. "He is our perfect bundle of sunshine." Chinooks, unfortunately, have nasty and unexpected side effects. They muddy streets and give people terrible headaches. Little did my parents realize that I embodied these gnarly aspects. My parents were going to be swept away by the gale-force wind that I would be.

You see, I was born autistic. No. Not the cliched kind of autistic people portrayed in pop culture. For starters, I am minimally speaking. I can't reliably communicate using speech. Unlike the autistic people conjured by Hollywood, I can neither beat Vegas nor deduce brilliant medical diagnoses out of thin air. My autism comes with a more specific set of quirks. An enduring love of videos of public transit. The ability to be entertained by math. A primal urge to smash drywall and dine on its spoils. A passion for poetry. A penchant for unbridled

Chapter 1: Chinook

aggression. A living and breathing theatre of Jekyll and Hyde. I am truly a force of nature. A natural phenomenon that is more the devil's handwork than God's. But every natural event needs a perfect storm of circumstances to come together. It doesn't happen overnight. What process shaped me into my current state? This is a self-exploration of how I got to where I am. A cautionary tale on how the education system can create storms like me. A manual on how not to treat powerless beings, whose only fault is being born with autism.

JANANI

ANANTHA'S FIRST TWO YEARS

Anantha means Eternal, one of the thousand names celebrating the Hindu God Vishnu, in a Sanskrit poem. From the beginning, we were drawn to that name. We looked at a thousand more names, perhaps even a thousand more, but kept returning to this one. It was a traditional name but also easy to pronounce.

When I was pregnant with Anantha, my husband and I did everything first-time expecting couples do. I read obsessively about anything pregnancy or delivery related. We went to multiple prenatal classes - one for a natural way of coping with childbirth called the Bradley method and another class offered by the hospital. I thought that getting the baby out was the most challenging part of pregnancy, but it turns out it wasn't. Anantha was born on a Saturday over Thanksgiving weekend. His labour and delivery were textbook perfect. The Bradley method helped with an unmedicated delivery, but things started going wrong once Anantha was delivered. I had a postpartum hemorrhage followed by an infection that required antibiotics for the next several days. Between my exhaustion and the demands of being a new mom, constantly

Chapter 1: Chinook

nursing and changing diapers, it felt like I had run into a brick wall.

When Anantha was a couple of weeks old, things took a turn for the worse. He started grunting in extreme discomfort after every feeding. He could not nurse for more than a minute or two. However, that meant he could not sleep for stretches longer than twenty minutes. If I was exhausted before, it was now multiplied several times over. The doctors couldn't help and assured us that it was colic, and that Anantha would outgrow the crying. The Internet frightened us, giving us multiple possibilities of truly terrible outcomes. I went on varied diets, eliminating gluten, dairy, and tomatoes, but nothing helped. This was not a pleasant, relaxing time. It is hard to relax and enjoy things when your baby is in obvious distress.

When Anantha was five months old, we went on a long airplane journey to India. Our trip there was a whirlwind of activity, where we went to the family temple at a place called Sholingur. We made the climb of over one thousand steps to behold the lord Narasimha and seek his blessings for all of us, especially the baby.

We returned from India when Anantha was a little over eight months old. My husband went back to work, and I stayed at home with Anantha, plunged into sudden loneliness, having no clue how to engage the baby. We went on occasional walks on the pathway, but, as I recall, it was a rainy summer with thunderstorms almost every day. My friends visited from Boston for a week with their toddler daughter, and we went to the zoo and Banff with both kids. It was a pleasant interlude in an otherwise blur of days where I mostly tried to get Anantha to eat or take a nap and failed miserably at both. I remember yelling at the bewildered little baby, frustrated at not having a moment for myself to do anything because he wouldn't even nap. I still cringe at the memory. I, of course, had no clue about sensory issues or anything else that might have contributed to Anantha's discomfort. I was too exhausted to have grace. A pattern that has repeated over and over through the years. I should have hired a babysitter or nanny for at least a couple of hours while I showered or napped, but hindsight is 20/20, and I was just a clueless first-time struggling mother.

I continued to meet with a few mothers from my prenatal class since we all had similar-aged babies. I remember the combined first birthday party; we did a cake smash. My son was one of the few who stood up and walked, and I was so proud. He hadn't crawled, but suddenly he was walking at almost one year of age. Despite my delight, I noticed that Anantha was quite different from the other babies. For example, I had also enrolled us in a mom and baby class, and I saw Anantha couldn't do many things other babies or toddlers were doing. I was concerned but tried to explain it away with, "That other baby is a whole month older. Next month, my son would be doing those things too." And a month later, I would still be confused but would somehow justify a missed milestone.

Mealtimes were also challenging. My son didn't like to eat and didn't like most food. Instead, Anantha would rock in his highchair, back and forth, hitting his head when we tried to feed him. This didn't seem normal, but

Chapter 1: Chinook

we didn't know if it warranted a trip to the doctor. We mentioned our concern at check-ups but were dismissed. Just like our fears about Anantha not talking! My son had less than ten words at eighteen months that didn't even sound clear. I remember going to the doctor in worry but was dismissed with the reply, "Boys take longer to talk."

Robert

MY CONNECTION TO AUTISM AND INCLUSIVE EDUCATION

I begin by sharing a little about my background and how my experiences have influenced how I think about and support Anantha in school. I hold a Bachelor of Arts degree specializing in Psychology and a Bachelor of Education degree specializing in Inclusive Education. Soon, I hope to obtain a master's degree in Special Education or Educational Leadership.

Early in my undergraduate studies, I began working at a residential facility for autistic youth aged six to eighteen. My work focused on teaching autistic children and youth to build independent living skills, communication skills, and regulation skills. Each autistic person I worked with was unique in how they communicated, moved, thought, and experienced the world around them- just like any other person. My early work placement also provided a real-world opportunity for me to see textbook theories in action. It is where I first learned how checklists of diagnostic criteria were used to label and categorize autistic people. I felt connected to the children and valued my work, however, my views were shaped by expectations

Chapter 1: Chinook

of normal ability based on diagnostic labels assigned by resident experts. Descriptions of the clients I worked with left me sometimes confused because they led to decisions that seemed contradictory to the autistic person's desires and interests-if acknowledged at all.

While working in a residential setting, I learned much about myself, including patience, the importance of being present, letting go of the small things, and the joy I felt when an autistic child learned a new skill. I was primarily humbled and wanted to know much more about autistic people. Once I completed my education degree in Inclusive Education, I was hired as a classroom teacher for students with developmental disabilities and complex behavioural challenges. Fast forward to my work with Anantha, where I worked as part of a team in a consultant-type role and provided mentorship and coaching to school staff to promote positive learning opportunities and positive classroom experiences for autistic students in inclusive settings.

I first met Anantha in the autumn of 2020. Chandra approached me to collaborate with the school to develop a plan for Anantha's transition to grade seven. As I read through the pages written by numerous professionals describing Anantha's bumpy educational past, I was intrigued. I wondered who this young man was and what story he had to tell. I was curious and driven to start the work.

To start planning for Anantha's back-to-school transition, the school team set up an initial meet and greet with me, Anantha, and his parents. I anxiously awaited this meeting, not entirely sure of what to expect. I arrived at the school and walked into the office. I was introduced to Janani and Diwakar, the school team (principal, assistant principal, teacher), and Anantha. I remember Anantha sitting in a chair in the office, twirling his fingers while his eyes darted around the room, anxiously taking everything and everyone in. He had a letter board on his lap, his primary mode of communication. His care worker was with Anantha, who helped him use his letter board to communicate. We decided it was best to walk down the hallway to the classroom. Diwakar and Janani remained in the office while I walked with Anantha, his care worker, and his teacher to what would be his grade seven classroom. I felt excited, and I remember thinking about how I imagined Anantha to be versus whom I saw in front of me. I realized I had worked him up to be something he was not. Like any other junior high student, he was in that awkward stage between child and young man.

During our brief meeting, Anantha's care worker helped Anantha participate in the conversation while his teacher asked questions. It was apparent how uncomfortable Anantha was during our meeting. I could see unsureness in his body language. His eyes darted around the room constantly. I thought about how overwhelming and strange this all must feel for Anantha. I wondered if we were asking too many questions and how much was too much, considering he was also processing the new classroom space. I introduced myself and said I was there to help Anantha be successful and feel included at school. I shared that I would be at the school each day he

Chapter 1: Chinook

attended, and I looked forward to getting to know him better. Through the support of Anantha's care worker and letter board, he shared that he was excited but worried about coming to school. I tried to reassure Anantha by stating that this was a normal feeling. We all agreed that Anantha could email and share things he was worried about, and we would all do our best to share our ideas and plans with him so that he didn't have to wonder what was in store for him at school. Toward the end of the meeting, Anantha asked, "When can I start school?" I smiled and said, "Right away, Anantha." His enthusiasm was inspiring.

As I walked out of the school and into my car, I felt my heart race. Ideas were rapidly flowing through my head about how to start the work and what my support might look like. I also felt something undeniable – Anantha was an extraordinary person. I felt connected and looked forward to getting to know him better. On the drive home, with a smile on my face, I called my coworkers and explained how the first meeting went. I was charged with excitement-I felt like I was meant to meet Anantha. The school team had different thoughts than mine, however. They were overwhelmed. On paper, Anantha is described as a semi-verbal autistic student, speaking only one or two words at a time. When Anantha speaks to communicate, the words he says do not necessarily correlate with the environment or conversations around him.

Anantha is typically in a constant state of hyperarousal, which is observed in his quick body movements, often closing his eyes, licking his fingers and other parts of his body, plugging his ears, rocking, and other motions when sitting or walking. Anantha checked all the typical autism boxes, which helped explain the bumpy educational path that led him in and out of various special, private, and public education placements. I could see that Anantha was greatly misunderstood. I suggested two goals to help the school frame the work before us. First, we would focus on learning about Anantha from his point of view; second, we would build a relationship with him. For Anantha to succeed at school, he needed to feel welcome and safe and know that his voice and perspective mattered.

Chandra

MY INTRODUCTION TO ANANTHA

Early in the school year of 2020, I received an email with several reports describing a complex autistic student who changed school placements yearly. This student, Anantha, was a semi-verbal autistic boy entering his first year of junior high school. Anantha's reports indicated that he was an English Language Learner with a moderate cognitive disability, mild delays in fine motor development, and significant difficulties with sensory processing, which caused him to be in a constant state of hyperarousal. Anantha's recent cognitive assessment indicated that his verbal comprehension was extremely high. He used a letter board and iPad to communicate with the support of a communication partner. The reports indicated that Anantha's skills ranged from extremely low to extremely high. With limited success, he attended special education classes, regular education classes, a private school, and home school.

The request was to review the documentation and work with the school to determine the appropriateness of Anantha attending a science-based school program. If so, how would this be possible? What would programming look like? Would he participate in full days? What support would be available? Would it be better for Anantha to start school in a special education class, then move to a mainstream class?

When I received the request, I was preparing to defend my doctoral research on inclusive best practices for autistic students. Fresh in my mind were all the studies, which, to be honest, were not more than two dozen, on the self-reported school experiences of autistic students. While limited, the results of these studies were exciting because they centred entirely on autistic students' perspectives. Which meant autistic students shared things that mattered most to them. While the views of parents and teachers are important, they can overshadow priorities identified by students. Absent from all the documentation I read was Anantha's voice. What was his opinion on his learning, ability, and responsive support?

Several conversations with team members followed to determine the steps we would take to support Anantha's return to school. There were moments within these conversations where I struggled to find the right words to express the options, I thought we could and should offer to Anantha because there was disagreement. I realized that there were very different ideas on inclusion for a mostly non-speaking autistic boy amongst us "experts." For example, beliefs about his physical participation in class varied. A few of my colleagues believed inclusion meant occasional integration into a mainstream class. For others, it meant that Anantha had to demonstrate his ability before having full access to a grade seven classroom.

Chapter 1: Chinook

When educators do not work from a common characterization of inclusion, it is challenging to identify shared goals and strategies to make meaningful student-centred inclusion happen. Inclusionary disagreement that leads to "fauxclusion" (Graham, 2020, p.7) isn't uncommon in schools, and without question, trickles down to students' everyday experiences. Several researchers have acknowledged this dissension. Framing it as, while most educators philosophically agree with the concept of equal education rights for all students, disparity exists in what this looks like day-to-day for students, especially students with significantly complex learner profiles like Anantha (Haug, 2017; Messiou, 2019; Mitchell & Sutherland, 2020).

Consequently, school jurisdictions have been criticized for becoming "masterpieces of rhetoric," leading to a "political oversell" (Haug, 2017, p. 207) that puts teachers in positions of unmanageability and failure. To help explain the disconnect between theory and practice, researchers have found that teachers and administrators lack the skill and confidence to support students with complex learning profiles (Domović, 2017; McCrimmon, 2015; Roberts & Webster, 2020; Tangen, 2005); and an increase in educational trends that value individualism, especially when governments make school funding contingent on student ability and performance (Haug, 2017).

INCLUSION: A PARTICIPATORY STUDENT EXPERIENCE

A common question asked by educators is, "What is inclusion?" Inclusion is a flexible, fluid, and iterative process guided by philosophies that value diversity, equity, acceptance, and belonging. If inclusion is thought of as a verb (action) as opposed to a noun (thing), we are better situated to frame inclusion as a participatory student experience (Graham, 2020). Framing inclusion as a participatory student experience conjures up words like student voice, self-advocacy, self-determination, autonomy, and opportunity. These actions also signify that the learning environment flexes to the abilities and needs of the student instead of the student conforming to the structures of the system. When inclusion is viewed as a participatory student experience, we can more precisely identify systemic structures and approaches that create barriers preventing the authentic inclusion of students with diverse abilities. Reframing the question from "What is inclusion?" to "In what ways can we be inclusive?" is a more productive starting point for educators as we seek ways to create meaningful learning and well-being experiences for students with disabilities in school.

CHAPTER 2: ELEVATORS

An Autistic Jump

Very intense are my joys.
Unlike the sober ones you enjoy.
I honour my special joy with an exalted jump upwards.
To commune with God
and thank him for my autism.
Alas, every jump inevitably brings me back to earth.
Good things sadly never last

~Anantha

Anantha

WHAT CANNOT BE LABELLED, CANNOT BE CURED

Elevators are a wondrous creation of mankind. Where others saw a prosaic invention of modern convenience, I discerned sheer poetry. Elevators seemed to welcome me with open arms while chiming the loveliest tunes. To me, they are a purveyor of heady sensory treats such as exhilarating movement, trippy lighting, and weird sounds. I yearned to be in their exalted company forever like star-crossed lovers. Alas, such love has many detractors. Romeo and Juliet didn't get to ride into the sunset. My attempts to woo the elevator by jumping to the sky while flapping my arms were met with stiff resistance from my very puzzled caregivers at daycare. They desperately tried to steer me to more "typical" activities. Blocks, rhymes, Lego, games - none of the routines appealed to my elevated heart. I was the boy without a user manual. Only, it was impossible to return or exchange me for someone more user-friendly!

Out of sheer confusion a plan was born to bell my eccentricities. The first step was to label myself. What cannot be labelled cannot be cured, you see. Apparently, I was in need of some serious curing. I was referred to

Chapter 2: Elevators

experts for a diagnosis. A diagnosis to discover my user manual and answer the puzzle I was.

JANANI

HIDDEN DIAGNOSIS

Sometime during the spring of 2009, when Anantha was one and a half years old, we went to the zoo as a family. This is my first memory of realizing that Anantha loved elevators. He didn't care about the animals. He would rush to the little glass viewing stations and stand expectantly, waiting for a non-existent door to close. At first, we didn't understand what he was doing. But over and over, he ran to similar-looking places, turned around, and brought his fingers together in front of his face, mimicking a closing door. An elevator!

In July of that same year, we moved to Northern Ireland for a few months. That was quite an adventure. A new place, new sights to see and new people in the apartment building we lived in. Weekends were fun since my husband was available, and the three of us would take a train to explore a different part of the country. Anantha fit into a tiny umbrella stroller, which was very convenient for travel, and he still mostly ate baby food. However, he discovered the yumminess of fries and pizza during those months. We went to many new places all over

Chapter 2: Elevators

Northern Ireland and even went on short trips to London and Edinburgh.

Weekdays were more challenging to find things to do for Anantha and me. We lived on the ninth floor with huge windows in our living room that looked to the streets below. Often, we would perch on the ledge, and I would point out cars to Anantha. We would also read books together; sometimes, I read aloud to Anantha and other times, he would look through books repeatedly on his own, as if he had an exam to study for. I went on long walks with Anantha, and often we would find our way to the mall or the pharmacy. On one of our walks, I discovered my son's next love- escalators. We rode up and down escalators incessantly and stopped only when I felt done, although Anantha never seemed to tire of them. When we visited City Hall or the Botanical Gardens, Anantha found his sources of enjoyment while I looked at flowers. For example, he was fascinated by the little hanging chains that kept people off the grass. Anantha would swing them back and forth and become absorbed in the patterns of light they created. Drains with their geometrical grates were another fascination for Anantha. He would bend over every single one we passed, studying them with intense concentration, though they all appeared the same to me.

Still in Ireland, I tagged along with a neighbour to a playgroup for toddlers. It was in a room inside a church. The moms were given tea, and the kids ran around the space with access to various toys and cookies. One of the organizers was a speech-language therapist who approached me afterward, saying, "Your son stuffed an entire cookie into his mouth." I wondered to myself, "Is this wrong? What kind of mother was I that I couldn't teach him how to eat a cookie properly? Was that a taught skill? How many such things would I have to teach?" I panicked and mumbled something apologetic about teaching him. "It could mean he has sensory issues. How's he doing with his speech?" Guilt came to me naturally and quickly. Sensory issues? What was that? Oh, he was delayed in his speech, and it was my fault because I didn't teach him to eat right! I was hyper-aware of my son's differences and how it was probably a reflection of my poor parenting. The therapist must have sensed my panic because she backed off, gently saying, "It's not a big deal. Just something to keep an eye on." I don't think I went to the playgroup again.

After a few months in Belfast, Anantha and I travelled to India to spend time with family. It was a good trip for the most part. Anantha was the apple of everyone's eye. He was suddenly talking much more, though he had an endearing sing-song way of speaking and often came up with his labels for things. For example, he called a fan "poovaada," which sounded quite exotic. He was loved and celebrated for everything he did or said, and he was happy. Anantha jumped and flapped his hands when he enjoyed something, and I remember my mother-in-law admiring this quality in Anantha. One exception was Anantha's second birthday party, a boisterous, noisy celebration with singing, music, and chatter. He looked miserable and spaced out.

Chapter 2: Elevators

We finally returned to Canada in December 2009, in the dead of winter in the middle of a snowstorm. I enjoyed my newfound freedom in India, where I had the time to think about working again. I had not intended to be a stay-at-home mom anyway and figured Anantha was old enough to start daycare. It might be good for him to be around other kids and for me to return to work. However, Anantha was miserable at daycare, and everyone reassured me that this was a typical response for young children. Anantha began attending daycare—a couple of hours, three times a week. "Why don't you increase the hours?" the staff asked. "He needs more time to get used to us. Short intervals like this only make it worse." I gradually lengthened Anantha's hours, but that didn't help. He became increasingly terrified of daycare. He became terrified if we even took the roads that might lead past the daycare to another destination. He became terrified of getting into the car lest we go to daycare. "Just a little bit of time at daycare," I would wheedle with him. This sentence has now permanently become one of Anantha's anxious stims. I could see Anantha's anxiety and how traumatic it was for him. My instincts were to pull him away, to put a stop to this. However, I didn't trust my instincts. Instead, I wondered if Anantha just needed a stronger parent. One who didn't crumble so quickly every time he crumbled. I saw the other kids thriving there, loving it, and playing happily. I kept hoping that Anantha needed more time to get used to the new environment. I persisted for a year and a half. It was a year and a half too long.

We attended early childhood music classes at Mount Royal University during that same time. It was sheer torture for Anantha because of the banging drums, varied tempos, and kids stomping their feet and clapping their hands. He would run to the doors, trying to escape. When Anantha found them locked, he would go into a frenzy, pulling down all the equipment, and maniacally opening and closing drawers. I look back at this now with a different lens, more aware of sensory dysregulation. At that time, though, I merely thought Anantha was being a naughty willful child and scolded him so much.

By the time Anantha was three, it was evident that he was very different from other kids. Our doctor still didn't see a reason for concern. I lamented about this one night to an acquaintance from my book club. I was giving her a ride, and somehow our conversation in the car ended up about my son. It turned out she was a social worker at a respite agency. She gave me the number of someone she knew. I called her contact and was told I could self-refer for an assessment at the Child Development Centre. This happened around October 2010. It would be almost another nine months before we got the actual assessment and Anantha's diagnosis of autism. During these months, I went from "What? My son can't possibly have autism! They're wrong!" to "Yes, my son does have autism. He checks so many of the boxes." Denial to acceptance is not an easy journey.

In those months, I had to acquire a lot of information. Suddenly, my reading was about developmental delays, therapies, autism, treatments, and cures. We saw a pediatrician in early 2011 who said she was sure he

Chapter 2: Elevators

had autism, even though she would wait for the formal assessment from the Child Development Centre before giving us an official diagnosis. Her manner was less than reassuring. Also, the doom and gloom narrative from the Internet sites I had been scouring meant I received the diagnosis badly. New acronyms like PUF (Program Unit Funding) and FSCD (Family Support for Children with Disabilities) began to dominate my conversations. I started seeking out other people with autistic children and stumbled on a mom's support group on Facebook specific to Calgary, Alberta. I lost most of my old friends anyway since my son was too different from their kids, and we were no longer welcome in their homes.

One new friend lent me a book, the first book I had read about autism. An intensely emotional book called *Let Me Hear Your Voice* by Catherine Maurice. I cried when I read it. The author finds salvation for her kids in ABA (Applied Behavioural Analysis), and towards the end of the book, her kids are in mainstream school, "indistinguishable from their peers." I would burn it if I got a copy of that book today. I certainly would never lend it to a parent of a newly diagnosed child. Alas, the clarity of hindsight. At that time, I drank the ABA Kool-Aid. Determined to help my child, I immersed myself in everything ABA. I had a goal now! I had to enroll my son in an ABA program, and my goal was that he would be mainstreamed in a school in a couple of years, and no one would even know that he was autistic! To that end, I didn't want to divulge the diagnosis to anyone, not even family. We went on another visit to India in the summer of 2011. Initially, we didn't let anyone know.

Robert

CHALLENGING ASSUMPTIONS AND PROVING ABILITY

While working with Anantha during the first few weeks at school, I realized that he was trying hard to prove to his teachers and classmates that he was a capable student who didn't belong in a segregated special education class. I think Anantha sensed that teachers and classmates wondered if he was capable of learning grade-level curriculum or even, because of his stimming and vocalizations, believed that he wasn't taking in information during lessons.

To help Anantha reduce the immense pressure he put on himself to prove to others that he was a capable student, I needed to find creative ways to make learning and social activities more accessible to Anantha so that he could focus on learning, not proving himself as capable. First, I wanted to find ways Anantha could still complete grade-level curriculum objectives, even when he attended school for less than two hours daily. Second, I wanted to ensure that Anantha felt socially connected to his peer group so that they would relate to Anantha based on similarities, not just differences. To set goals in both these

Chapter 2: Elevators

areas, I knew that Anantha needed frequent access to gross motor and sensory activities to regulate his body. Having regular, non-contingent access to hallways, the gymnasium, and the sensory room meant that Anantha could respond to his body whenever he felt he needed to. I knew that scheduling his regulation would never work and that his internal states were much more fluid, which meant we had to be too. Because Anantha needed frequent sensory breaks, it was also essential to reassure Anantha that taking these breaks was okay and that he did not have to try and pretend or mask his needs to feel like he belonged at school. We needed to reassure Anantha that he could be in school in ways that supported his needs without fear of judgment or that he was a burden.

During these first few months, Anantha helped me rethink how teachers show our students that we welcome and respect their diversity. One of the best ways to do this is through the accommodations we provide for them. We use theories and words like differentiation, personalization, universal design for learning, and so on, but sometimes it feels like we are just checking a box. The teacher workload is hefty and increasingly complex, so I understand how our good intentions get lost in the busyness and demands of the day. We need to find a better way to walk the talk, however. How can we use school-wide approaches to support teachers and students?

An example of all-inclusive thinking is when Anantha shared his design ideas for school playgrounds. The class assignment was for students to design different ways school playgrounds could be more enjoyable for students. Anantha shared that having stimulating and calming equipment would appeal more to students like him because it would help him feel less socially anxious or physically overwhelmed. Anantha suggested that having a series of tunnels that filtered bright lights, and sounds would provide more calming activities for autistic students to enjoy at recess. Anantha's peers were impressed with his ideas and rationale and asked detailed questions to learn more about Anantha's design ideas. At the core of Anantha's response to his peers was to include the perspectives of neurodiverse students in the planning process and for adults to be open to student feedback.

My personal view on inclusion was most impacted when Anantha shared his response to a writing assignment I gave to him on a day he was participating in school from home. I asked Anantha, "List five ways to win your heart – what can someone do to get you on their side?" Anantha wrote back:

> *Treat me respectfully by presuming my competence.*
> *Include me in regular classrooms with meaningful support for my disability.*
> *Use positions of power to help people like me instead of crushing our dreams.*
> *Stop asking us to prove ourselves repeatedly… education is a fundamental human right.*
> *Treat me with honey-dipped donuts from Tim Hortons.*

Chapter 2: Elevators

It was clear to me that, every day, Anantha was fighting for his right to be included in school. It was impossible not to get behind him and ride that elevator.

Chandra

REVISITING THE HISTORY OF AUTISM

The diagnostic labelling and subsequent treatment of autistic people do not occur in a vacuum but are influenced by several factors, including history and politics. Revisiting earlier narratives on autism is helpful because we can better understand why over time, some forms of knowledge are revered more than others. Which, for autistic people, has meant that they have experienced years of misrecognition, harmful treatment, and exclusion.

The history of autism is commonly presented in the work of Eugen Bleuler, who, in 1910, described the concept of autism as a withdrawal from the external world and a symptom of schizophrenia (Greydanus & Toledo-Pereya, 2012; Verhoeff, 2013). Bleuler's definition of autism, based on the derivative of the Greek word autos, meaning self (Merriam-Webster, 2020), reflected a different way of thinking observed in autistic individuals (Frith, 1991). Bleuler's theories on autistic thinking questioned the legitimacy of human ability in relation to the psyche and linked medicalized definitions of ability and disability to autism.

Chapter 2: Elevators

In the 1930s, Austrian pediatrician, eugenicist and medical professor Hans Asperger published research on what he termed autistic psychopathy (Frith, 1991). Asperger's description of autistic characteristics included "a lack of empathy, little ability to form friendships, one-sided conversations, intense absorption in a special interest, and clumsy movements" (Attwood, 1997, p. 11). Asperger also noted literal-mindedness, anxiety, high speaking ability and, in some instances, intellectually giftedness (Bergenmar et al., 2015). Eventually, the term high-functioning autism became synonymous with Asperger's Syndrome. In one of Asperger's 1939 case studies, Asperger describes interactions between a boy and his mother. Anchoring a portion of his analysis on his belief that women are usually more "emotional than intelligent" (Frith, 1991, p. 41), Asperger concludes that the boy and his mother were equally strange. While Asperger's work mainly remained unnoticed in the English-speaking world until Lorna Wing translated from German to English in the 1980s (Wing, 1981).

In 1943 Austrian American psychiatrist and physician Leo Kanner introduced a new psychiatric condition called early infantile autism (Verhoeff, 2013). Kanner distanced himself from Bleur's theories of autism (as a feature of adult schizophrenia), instead believing autism to be a psychobiological disorder influenced by biological, psychological, and social factors (Eisenberg & Kanner, 1956, p.564). As a result of Kanner's research, the boundaries of autism expanded to include language and perceived cognitive abnormalities (Verhoeff, 2013). Kanner's theory on the psychobiological origins of autism also inferred controversial parental causation theories, including maternal coldness and a lack of affection (Eisenberg & Kanner, 1956; Kotsopoulos, 2014). In 1948, Time Magazine published an article on Kanner's work titled *Medicine: Frosted Children* (Time Magazine, April 26, 1948), describing autistic children as "diaper-aged schizoids" and their parents as "cold perfectionists" (Time Magazine, 1948, para. 3; Waltz, 2005). Time Magazine concluded their article with the question, "Were the cold parents freezing their children into autism?" (Donavan & Zucker, 2016, p. 79). Thus, inferring parents, known as refrigerator mothers (Donvan & Zucker, 2016), was responsible for causing their child's autism. The broad impact of Time Magazine's publication on families, particularly mothers of autistic children, was damaging, to say the least. Families were publicly blamed for their child's perceived abnormalities, and mothers were expected to undergo psychotherapy as part of their child's remediation (Chamak, 2008; Kotsopoulos, 2014). Kanner's inclusion of language and cognitive differences to identify autism served to exclude autistics from normative categories more precisely and consistently. Autistic children were commonly categorized according to their "devalued difference" (Goodley et al., 2014, p. 347) or strange ability; either way, they deviated from typical categories of human functioning (Saur & Sidorkin, 2018).

In 1967, Austrian-American Bruno Bettelheim published an article titled *Infantile Autism: The Birth of Self*. In it, he writes of a boy whom he describes as a "boy-machine," "a robot," and a "machine powered body" who has built up his defences to protect himself from his refrigerator mother (Zager et al., 2012). Standardized medical or psychological tests have not substantiated Bettelheim's theories on autism (Waltz, 2005). They have since been discredited based on evidence of falsification of academic credentials, plagiarism, and the mistreatment of children (Greydanus & Toledo-Pereyra, 2012). While Bettelheim's contributions to theories and treatment of autism have been discredited, history cannot unknow his philosophies and the fact that they represented extreme and sometimes violent theories of ability, difference, and what it means to be human.

AUTISM RESEARCHERS IN THE CONTEXT OF NAZI GERMANY

As previously mentioned, theories about autism and (mis) perceptions of autistic ability do not exist in a vacuum but instead live in connection to broader social and political contexts. In recent years attention has been placed on the patriarchs of autism and their connection to and influence from Nazi Germany. Hence, it is relevant to point out the political powers that shaped Asperger, Kanner and Bettelheim's education and life experiences; and how these likely contributed to modern ideas and treatment of autistic people. For instance, all three men were born in Austria between 1894 and 1906. Kanner and Asperger each served in the German army, with Kanner serving in World War I and Asperger serving in World War II

(Neumärker, 2003). Bettelheim was imprisoned for ten months in a concentration camp, and after the war, he and Kanner immigrated to the United States (Greydanus & Toledo-Pereyra, 2012). Asperger and Bettelheim reportedly censored parts of their histories to protect and legitimize their professional identities. For instance, Asperger was accused of sending disabled children to be euthanized during World War II (Hippler & Klicpera, 2003; Scheffer, 2018). Bettelheim misrepresented his background and credentials to secure university professorial and director positions (Pollack, 1997).

In her book titled *Asperger's Children: The Origins of Autism in Nazi Vienna*, Scheffer (2018) highlights the Third Reich "as a diagnosing regime... obsessed with sorting the population into categories, cataloguing people by race, politics, religion, sexuality, criminality, heredity, and biological defects" (p.18), which ultimately shaped Asperger's theory of autism. In addition to Sheffer, other scholars have questioned the legitimacy of society's reverence for the patriarchs of autism. As more publications became translated into English, evidence emerged that autism research existed before Asperger's and Kanner's work. For instance, it has been suggested that Asperger may have known about a female Russian scientist, Grunya Sukhareva's 1925 publication describing features of autism that are very similar to current DSM-5 descriptions of autism (Zeldovich, 2018). However, Asperger may have avoided crediting Sukhareva's work because she was Jewish and a woman who was likely not favoured by the Third Reich (Zeldovich, 2018). Without dispute,

Chapter 2: Elevators

Europe's political and social landscape during the first half of the 21st century was fraught with oppressive and conformist ideologies that permeated the thinking of prominent scientists, which unquestionably influenced our current medical, social, and educational beliefs on difference, disability, belonging, and inclusion.

CHAPTER 3: CONVERSION

Ode to a Therapist

If you really knew me...
Beneath the cloak of apathy.
Beyond the armour of anger.
Buried within the mounds of stims.
Bubbling below the sea of angst.
Bright rests a mirror.
Beseeching you to
Behold the you in me.

~Anantha

Anantha

REMEDIATING AUTISM

"Your autistic son needs very intensive conversion therapy," asserted the autism expert. "We will aggressively modify him, so he becomes normal. He can avail himself of a life as a productive human. Applied Behaviour Analysis (ABA) has transformed the lives of so many families like yours." My hapless parents were utterly sold on ABA. And so began my conversion, Anantha Krishnamurthy, the yet unproductive and savage autistic.

ABA works on the sacred mantra of rewarding typical behaviours and punishing autistic ones. I was studied for hours to identify rewards that made me dance to ABA's tune. The cheese was not just a snack, you see. It was a potent weapon to stop my calming stims. God, forbid I enjoy reading for the sheer intrinsic joy of it. No, cheese had to be a treat I got for something as inane as staying still during my session. These types of idiotic strategies continued relentlessly. I started revolting. The ABA pundits responded every time with heavier artillery. My parents watched in horror, helplessly caught in the crossfire.

ABA mercilessly crushed my sense of worth under the cloak of "rigorously peer-reviewed" therapy. It constantly

Chapter 3: Conversion

made me hate my autism and hence by extension myself. My conversion was well and truly complete when my parents pulled the plug off ABA. I went from a sweet kid filled with wonder and curiosity (and love of elevators) to a violent, self-loathing and anxious wreck. And I hated cheese and reading.

The quest for my user manual continued.

Janani

THE JOURNEY THROUGH EARLY INTERVENTION, PRE-SCHOOL, AND KINDERGARTEN

When we travelled again to India in 2011, my son was loved and celebrated by all our family and friends. However, some things stood out now that he was older. One morning I went downstairs to see him near the gate, flapping and jumping, surrounded by many kids on the other side who laughed mockingly at Anantha. I was heartbroken. Is this how other kids would treat my son throughout his life? While he was happy to be in India, the sheer assault on his senses in terms of sounds, smells, and unpredictable schedules left him crying inconsolably. Our families were perplexed by his rapid mood changes from happy one minute to uncontrollably crying the next. At some point, I broke down and told them his diagnosis. We were initially met with disbelief, denial, and anger at the medical professionals giving Anantha this label. There was also some subtle blaming about my inability to parent or not providing proper intellectual nourishment for Anantha.

Little was known about autism in India at that time. What little they knew, they equated it with people who had an intellectual disability. "Look, he is so intelligent!" was a common refrain among family members anytime Anantha labelled something or said something cute. Anantha would start preschool when we returned to Calgary in September of that same year. The therapy model in Alberta for young kids diagnosed with autism was twofold. They would attend a preschool program for part of the day, and for the other part of the day, they would have therapy at home for two to three hours, depending on the agency.

PRE SCHOOL

We were told by professionals, other parents, and our family support worker that our only option for a preschool placement was one of the few specialized preschools in the city. A few agencies supported kids in regular preschools, but this option was for "higher functioning" kids, a phrase used to indicate how fluently a child spoke. For the first year of his preschool, Anantha attended a well-known specialized preschool with branches throughout the city. After all the trauma of daycare, I was worried that Anantha would also hate preschool. To my surprise, he seemed to be reasonably happy attending. They had minimal expectations, but they allowed the kids to relax and explore, and there were some kind staff members.

HOME THERAPY AND APPLIED BEHAVIOURAL ANALYSIS (ABA)

Our home therapy was with an Applied Behavioural Analysis (ABA) agency. The contrast between home therapy and school was striking. Our first aide was a lovely young woman who has remained in touch with us. She had a list of teaching programs typically used when a child starts ABA therapy. This included imitating gestures, imitating block patterns, identifying items, and categorizing groups of objects. She also used a token board to reward Anantha's desired behaviour. For every five things Anantha did correctly, he received a reward. Most of his rewards included tickles, songs, and airplane rides, where she carried him around, making a "whooshing" sound. Anantha seemed to love it and adored her! He was making great progress, and I remember the program coordinator saying how much she loved Anantha and how compliant he was and wishing she could clone him for her caseload. An odd compliment, but at that time, I didn't understand the implicit messaging behind her comment. I merely smiled in pride.

In the first few months of ABA therapy, Anantha enjoyed the novelty of the program and the intellectual excitement of learning new concepts. Our first aide quit in a couple of months because she was moving away, and we got replacement aides from the agency. They were nice women, both well-trained, but they blindly followed protocol instead of trying to think of new activities. Most of the program was based on DTT (Discrete Trial Training)

Chapter 3: Conversion

and involved repeated trials of the same task. This meant that Anantha had to complete ten trials of repeating block patterns and get 8 of 10 correct to move on to the next step. An 80% achievement goal was considered mastery, which in theory, made sense. Practically though, Anantha was incredibly bored when he got to the sixth trial of the teaching activity. Therefore, Anantha would lose interest and not achieve the 80% criteria and would have to repeat the task again and again. I could see the problem and suggested they lower the threshold. My requests were not heard until the team meetings. The aides themselves were too unmotivated or powerless to make such changes. I was not vocal enough then. If I am more vocal these days in my advocacy, it's because I've had years of not being heard (resulting in regret) as my training.

I remember one incident where the aide had a big plastic bin of animal figurines for Anantha to sort into categories. Another teaching task repeated ad nauseum. As she pulled out the animals one by one, Anantha identified each one, some of whom I didn't know the names myself. He identified about 99 animals! I was so impressed. I looked at the aide, thinking she would be similarly impressed. She merely looked bored since it was not part of the program anyway, and we were wasting time.

Team meetings happened monthly, where a whole group of professionals ranging from the program directors and coordinators, sat around the room with Anantha in the centre. In his presence, the team talked about Anantha treating him like a lab animal. I was part of the circle, too, though my role was limited to asking occasional questions. The professionals loved to hear their voices and could go on and on. I cringe to remember this time and cannot begin to fathom the extent of trauma this created in Anantha. He was an intellectual curiosity to his team, not a human child worthy of respect and dignity. Once a month, we had access to a speech-language therapist and an occupational therapist who worked in our home and added some programs of their own to the ever-expanding list. The occupational therapist mostly worked on self-help skills like dressing and eating. She was good and efficient. However, some of the things we were asked to do, like withholding cheese from his apples and cheese snack, came from her reasoning on building motivation and compliance in him. Anantha had to take four or five bites of non-preferred food to access the food reward. Eventually, he liked fewer and fewer foods instead of expanding his repertoire. This pattern was repeated across all areas of teaching. The rewards that Anantha was initially motivated to work for became less and less motivating for him. Toys that he liked were no longer interesting. It became harder and harder to find reinforcers. Anantha used to love books, but they became a part of a torturous program of joint attention. If everything you love is held as ransom or proof of your imperfection, it's easy to give up.

Eventually, Anantha started acting up. The "perfect compliant child" was now resisting therapy, more anxious, and showed signs of poor self-esteem. If rewards were not motivating, perhaps their absence would work, at least in managing his behaviour. The team modified

Chapter 3: Conversion

his programming so he would earn tokens but quickly lose them because he yelled or spit or threw the blocks. Eventually, it became more difficult for Anantha to earn rewards. One more reason to give up since the promised reward was practically unattainable, and who knew if he could hold it together until then! There was no distinguishing between "can't" and "won't." Everything was seen as voluntary behaviour. I saw a hopeless, anxious child, dysregulated, unable to do or say much except protest in ways he knew how. At the time, we were painted a picture of Anantha, by professionals, as a stubborn, willful child who delighted in using his intelligence only in maladaptive ways. We sincerely believed we were doing the best for our son through all this work- and we gave it our all. We volunteered at casinos, roasted hot dogs, and begged businesses for silent auction items to support funding for the agency we partnered with.

Most people say they don't want to change their children. They merely want to teach them so that they can adapt to this world better. We would have said the same. We certainly believed it. However, every one of our goals on the Individual Student Plan (ISP) was ableist. Most of the goals centred around more speech and playing and socializing with peers in typical ways. For example, one of the goals was to address Anantha's bug phobia. He was terrified of flying insects such as flies, bees, and wasps. The responding therapy consisted of giving candy to Anantha every time he did not react in fear to the bugs. In the short term, he learned to mask his fear. It did nothing to address the fear itself in the long term, and Anantha is still scared of bugs all these years later. The program director got a nice academic paper from her work, which allowed her to graduate from her master's program.

Our home therapy team had convinced us that inconsistency in therapy styles was confusing my son. They kept hammering home the urgency of intense therapy right away before "the window of opportunity" closed. The theory was that maximum progress would be obtainable before a child turned six years old. Now my son was in an ABA program full-time, and they promised us that we'd see amazing progress. I drove across town to take my son to his preschool and therapy appointments. I was pregnant with my daughter, which was tiring—a small sacrifice in my mind for the greater good. Things didn't get better; they got worse in some ways. Anantha became more anxious, and anxiety management crept into ISP goals. Anantha's team didn't believe in sensory and dysregulation issues because all behaviour functions were viewed as maladaptive! The only tool used to manage Anantha's anxiety was a laminated book with the alphabet, which he was expected to flip through slowly while reading each letter aloud. We had a very non-compliant, angry child who would spit in defiance by the end of his preschool year. Withholding his iPad seemed to be the only motivator that somewhat worked, but even it was fraught with many meltdowns.

I felt sick whenever I told Anantha he couldn't have his iPad. I remember his little tear-stained face, desperately screaming, "sorry!" If I relented and gave in, he would huck the iPad across the room. There was no winning.

We became the parents who could not control our child and were receiving scorn from others, who thought we were too soft! Even other parents of autistic kids seemed shocked every time my son acted up.

KINDERGARTEN

In 2013, after much deliberation on where to enroll Anantha in kindergarten, we decided to go with a community group-run kindergarten program that would allow our ABA aide to accompany him. The idea was that she would assist him with things he found difficult while he was exposed to a typical educational setting. It was meant to be a gentle introduction to a regular classroom. Instead, the aide ran a parallel classroom in the hallway, trying to enforce compliance. Anantha was not allowed in the classroom until he could sit still, listen and be typical, even though the last criteria was unspoken. Within a month of Anantha starting kindergarten, he was kicked out. The teacher said she rarely saw him and didn't feel like he was her student. When we came out of the long and challenging meeting (with Anantha present), the program director of the ABA agency had the gall to blame the failure on Anantha not being motivated enough. We used candy as reinforcers, but they no longer worked. "What else does he like? How about his morning hot chocolate? Let's make that conditional on good behaviour." I was startled. The hot chocolate was meant to be nutritious, especially since Anantha was not big on breakfast; it wasn't meant to be used as a reward. Seeing my hesitation, she reiterated,

"We have to hit him where it hurts, Janani." Those exact words, spoken about a five-year-old child, were the last straw. I held my rage all the way home, determined to cut ties with this toxic agency.

Anantha had to stay home for a month while I figured out our options. We felt he still wasn't ready for public school and wanted to give him more time in a protective setting. Therefore, we chose a different non-ABA-based specialized kindergarten program for Anantha. More driving around town while my baby girl napped in the car's back seat! We thought we were free of ABA and the future was nothing but bright. We could not have been more wrong. The tyranny of low expectations was waiting around the corner.

Robert

RECONCEPTUALIZING TIME AND SPACE TO SUPPORT INCLUSION

One of the first ideas we collaborated with Anantha on was to rethink traditional ideas of time and space to allow him to communicate, engage in learning, and interact with peers in ways that respect his unique sensory profile. During the first few months of school, Anantha gradually increased his school attendance from short visits after school hours to half days during school hours. The time he was in school may have seemed short and unmeaningful to some, but I knew that Anantha was using all his energy to keep his body regulated and to concentrate on learning. By rethinking time and space specific to Anantha, he was gradually able to increase his attendance at school. This accommodation meant Anantha could use different learning spaces like the learning commons across the hall from his classroom, sensory room, and gymnasium. Having a space directly across from the classroom was beneficial because it allowed Anantha to gradually enter the busy classroom when he decided it suited him. Time and space were controlled by Anantha, not by bells and schedules. As Anantha's anxiety lessened, I could see him opening up to his teacher and classmates.

To support Anantha's transition to more extended periods in the classroom, we agreed that he would have complete choice and control to go for a walk or access different school spaces whenever he needed to. It is interesting how much more we made learning accessible to Anantha when we altered how he used space and time at school. Accommodations about time and space did not require specialized theories or training. Our modifications and strategies were effective because they were created together with Anantha, and we leveraged existing opportunities within the school. Anantha gradually learned to trust that his voice would be included in identifying goals and strategies and that his school team wanted what was best for him. This trusting relationship helped reduce Anantha's anxiety at school. Essentially, Anantha knew we had his back and that his voice and choice would consistently be honoured. After all, he knew what worked best for him and when changes needed to be made.

There were several instances where Anantha's school team created terrific opportunities for Anantha to show his deep knowledge of the subject matter by flexing time and space. I vividly remember a time when Anantha's English teacher shared with the class Anantha's book review. Anantha pre-recorded text-to-voice audio messages and submitted them to his teacher so that he could contribute to a class discussion. Anantha's peers were struck by Anantha's insightful responses and were introduced to new ideas on inclusion, ableism, and politics. The

Chapter 3: Conversion

conversation among Anantha's peers was energized and inquisitive. Anantha glowed from the positive attention and affirmations he received from his peers and teacher. Once the class discussion ended, Anantha told me he wanted to take a break. Together we walked to the sensory room. Anantha was visibly happy, flapping his hands and bouncing his body while rocking back and forth. Anantha seemed to reflect on his classroom experience during our time in the sensory room. Immediately after taking a break, Anantha and I talked through a few of his classmate's questions and started to record some responses on his iPad. Anantha continued to respond to his classmates from home, but before he left, he typed, "I feel great and had an amazing day!"

Because teachers have had to learn to pivot between online and in-class teaching during the pandemic, we have become more open to the idea that learning can be meaningful and interactive outside of the "bums in seats" type of thinking. When Anantha is not in class, his virtual attendance is supported by communication logs with teachers and chat forums to connect with classmates about assignments and group projects. Offering hybrid learning spaces has been a crucial strategy to help Anantha because it has reduced the pressure on Anantha to conform to traditional ideas of participation and inclusion. It also allows his school team and Anantha to make micro-adjustments to support his sensory needs without fear of being judged.

Chandra

DEINSTITUTIONALIZATION TO INCLUSION

Institutionalized care was recommended by doctors, suggesting that for severely autistic children to become less autistic, they should be removed from the influences of parents and home (Chamak, 2008; Chomer, 2014). Like many other institutionalized children with disabilities, autistic children experienced experimental and unethical treatments, including lysergic acid diethylamide (LSD). This hallucinogenic drug causes alterations in thoughts, feelings, and awareness, including seeing and hearing things that do not exist (National Institute of Drug Abuse, 2016). Researchers hypothesized that LSD treatments would promote speech, and electric shock treatments would reduce problem behaviour in autistic children (Kirkham, 2017; Sigafoos et al., 2007).

The deinstitutionalization of disabled children was influenced by lobbyists' work, including parent advocates, who defended that all children had a right to live at home and receive a public education (Donovan & Zucker, 2016). Until the mid-1970s in the United States, a school jurisdiction had the authority to refuse education if a child was considered ineducable. Ruth Sullivan, a mother of an autistic child, was one of the leading lobbyists for *The Education for All Handicapped Children*, now known as *The Individuals with Disabilities Education Act* (IDEA) (Wood, 2016). IDEA legislates that all students with disabilities in the United States receive a Free and Appropriate Public Education. According to a report published by the Canadian Centre for Policy Alternatives (Towle, 2015), a child's right to access free education is protected by several international laws, including *The Convention on the Rights of the Person with Disability* (United Nations in Convention on the Rights of Persons with Disabilities, 2006) and guidelines such as the *Salamanca Statement and Framework for Action on Special Needs Education* (UNESCO, 1994); however, Canada has no federal legislation mandating a disabled child's right to inclusive education. Instead, the regulation of inclusive education falls under each province and territory (Towle, 2015).

REMEDIATION AND CURE

Ole Ivar Lovaas, a clinical psychologist from UCLA, also believed that autistic children could be taught "normalized" behaviours using Applied Behavioural Analysis [ABA] (Lovaas & Buch, 1977). Theories of ABA arose from behavioural psychology in the 1910s (Kirkham, 2017) and was first used to condition animals' behaviour, as famously recognized in the work of BF. Skinner (Kirkham, 2017). Principles of behaviourism were first applied to autistic children in the 1960s, and Lovaas was considered the pioneer of using behaviour modification, including punishments, to cure autistic children of their autism. Lovaas reported that when autistic children received a minimum of 40 hours per week of ABA therapy, approximately 47% achieved normal functioning, 43% made significant progress, and 10% made little progress (Kirkham, 2017; Sallows & Graupner, 2005). However, researchers have disputed these findings arguing a weak methodology, insignificant effect sizes, and no statistically significant differences between outcomes of students who participated in special education programs for non-speaking students and those who participated in the Lovaas method (Ospina et al., 2008). Lovaas' ABA program was made available to parents through his book *Teaching Developmentally Disabled Children: The Me Book* (Lovaas, 1981), but was criticized by other scientists and parents for the inhumane use of aversives, also called punishments for incorrect responses made by autistic children (Kirkham, 2017).

While many parents and allies questioned the ethical treatment of autistic children who participated in ABA programs, medical and community experts offered few alternatives. In response to intense scrutiny by disability advocates, traditional ABA programs have since softened their approaches. However, many researchers and scientists continue to believe that the benefits of conventional ABA have been exaggerated (Fernell et al., 2015; Weiss & Delmolino, 2006) and that initial claims of effectiveness and cure have not been replicated (Matson & Neal, 2012). Furthermore, many autistic self-advocates strongly view the principles and practices of ABA to be abusive and unethical (Chamak, 2008; Gruson-Wood, 2016; Socially Anxious Advocate, 2015) and that it "takes away our voice" (Bascom, 2012, p.182). Like Anantha, autistic advocate Ido Kedar (2018) recalls ABA therapy as a time of suffering and that he continues to get PTSD flashbacks just hearing the phrases "High Five!" and "Good Job!" (Kedar, 2018, para. 2).

GROWTH MINDSET

From the beginning of my career, I was trained in the principles of ABA and used them for years. Admittedly I was intrigued by the theory, and the concrete thinker in me liked the highly structured, sequential pedagogy and the copious amounts of data-keeping. However, there were times when deep down, something felt off to me when I used this method to teach my autistic students. One day, I formulaically presented the blocks, gave the direction or S^D (discriminative stimulus) to "give me the number 5 block", and was quick to deliver a prompt if the student took too long to respond, looked away, or even touched their nose before responding (in case the student inadvertently learned to associate their nose with the number 5 if I didn't intervene). When the student answered correctly, I gave them a reinforcer, usually a tiny piece of candy. I then cleared the materials from the desk to signal that the trial was over, and then I would prepare for the subsequent trial. This pattern continued for the entire school day, day after day. This morning, as I set the timer to 3-minutes and told the student to take a break from the desk we both occupied, I noticed something in his eyes when he turned away from me. His big brown eyes looked beyond sad-they looked utterly defeated.

I am unsure why this thought came to me so quickly, but I instantly thought, "I just put out his light." It was a weighty moment for me where curriculum, pedagogy and evidence of mastery superseded human connection and care. Like so many teachers, I truly cared for this little boy and wanted so much for him because I saw so much ability and potential. This was the moment when a significant shift in my teaching mindset occurred. From then on, I focused less on prioritizing teaching targets and assessments and listened more to students' spoken and unspoken words. And when I listened, I also watched. I watched my autistic students for instances of curiosity, moments of joy, and feelings of frustration and sadness. I watched for learning activities and spaces they moved towards and away from, which meant I watched for opportunities to teach and moments to let them be - themselves. Instead of pathologizing their autistic characteristics, I made space for them, meaning I accepted them.

Ever since I could remember, I have wanted to be a teacher, and I loved every aspect of my challenging job. However, despite my eagerness and passion as a beginning teacher, I wasn't yet confident in my skills, nor was I experienced enough to question the integrity of the curriculum or the methods I used to teach. There are moments in every teacher's classroom where experts and theories aside, the path forward is evident when we view

Chapter 3: Conversion

the student and situation from an unassuming, student-centred, and strength-based lens. What person, let alone a young child, would ever be motivated to get out of bed every morning to be subjected to multiple learning experiences that aim to remediate? To work each day to be less of themselves and be more "normal." Sometimes, I wonder if, in our thirst for evidenced-based success to support students with disabilities, we have educated ourselves out of common sense and forgotten the critical importance of ensuring acceptance, belonging, and human connection in education.

CHAPTER 4: HOLES

The Placement

Warm winds of the western ghats.
Whistling a winsome winter tune.
A luxuriant sensual soak.
Prying away the sun's sultry embrace.
Tropical fragrances.
Unleashing an olfactory tsunami.
The mighty midsection mumbles.
Cooking up grand post spa escapades.
A buffet at the farmer's field.
A stint as Ganesha's alter ego.
Trading blessings for coconuts.
Lording over heaven.
Whoosh!
The arctic air downs the curtain.
Show is over!
Freud is a fraud!
What a meaningless dream.
For an elephant in Edmonton.

~Anantha

Anantha

THE PROBLEM WITH AUTISM EXPERTS

My inclusion in a regular classroom was good therapy from the scars of ABA. It was a relief learning real things instead of participating as a lab rat in pointless ABA experiments. I had a kind education assistant who helped regulate me when autism got intense on me. My teacher, by virtue of not being an autism expert, was open to the fact that I could learn grade-level lessons.

The autism experts, though, cut my dream again. "He seems retarded," they essentially said, using a lot of psychological jargon to sugar-coat their diagnosis. "Educating him is a futile undertaking," they conveyed with the absolute certainty that fancy degrees seem to bestow on people. "He would benefit from a placement that teaches life skills like tying shoelaces," they declared, banging the metaphorical gavel on my hopes and dreams.

Several holes emerged because of the decision to deny me an education. The biggest one was the logical hole that equated not speaking with not thinking. You see, I perfectly knew the answers to every single question on the psych assessment test that earned me a life skills placement. My broken autistic body lacked the ability to

Chapter 4: Holes

translate my brain's instructions to either spoken or written format. This possibility was never entertained, leaving a gaping hole in my psyche. Psychological holes led to physical ones on my parents, aides, and their belongings.

Janani

NAVIGATING BUREAUCRATIC SYSTEMS

As I sit down to write this, I have a mental image of my child, all of six years old, clad in battered armour, going forth to meet increasingly Herculean challenges. I want to hug that child and beg his forgiveness. Childhood shouldn't have to be so complicated and traumatic. It shouldn't have been a daily battle with unknown foes.

THE FIRST DAY OF SCHOOL

In 2013 I remember the initial meeting at the specialized school that Anantha was to attend for kindergarten. The intake manager showed us around, and I could see Anantha trying hard to show off all he knew! He wanted to impress her by saying aloud words like "car" and "Calgary." She wasn't paying much attention to him, but I was. My heart ached for him, but I didn't know how I could help him. This was symptomatic of how he would be treated at school and elsewhere over the coming years. I remember laughing when the intake person asked me if my son was aggressive. "Not at all!" I said proudly. I had to eat my words when he bit his teacher hard enough

Chapter 4: Holes

to draw blood at the end of the first week. Anantha was labelled as a problem child with "behaviours," and we were referred to a psychologist in the school. I still don't know what the psychologist did apart from giving us stacks of photocopied handouts about generic topics on autism.

My husband and I took turns observing Anantha at school for a morning. Neither of us was happy with what we saw. I saw indifferent staff trying to get through the day. The kids who spoke well got all the attention and teaching. The others had to be kept busy somehow. I remember Anantha being handed a puzzle of American Sign Language (ASL) symbols and told to complete it. The sheer panic on his face as he tried to match the pictures to the letters prompted me to ask if he had done it before. He hadn't! Had they taught this in class before? No. Then why was Anantha expected to do something completely new without instruction or assistance? "Oh, it's just something to keep him busy. He likes this sort of thing," the education assistant replied.

Once, my husband observed Anantha at play outdoors and how he kept trying to escape the overwhelming noise of the playground by bolting. At one point, a menacing-looking man blocked his way and hollered at him, startling him into not bolting. My husband took a video of the interaction on his cellphone, and we used it to file a complaint. We were reprimanded for illegally recording a video on school premises.

HOME THERAPY TEAM

Things with our home team were no better. We put together a private team of professionals, many of whom charged twice or thrice reimbursed rates. I knew I didn't want ABA, but I didn't know what would help Anantha. I was still floundering around, trying to figure out what was best for Anantha. I kept hearing about Son-Rise and DIRFloortime® as a child-friendly approach to therapy. I was still trapped in the paradigm of believing that Anantha needed to play and socialize in typical ways. Son-Rise didn't seem accessible to us unless I planned to spend a small fortune and travel to Massachusetts for training. Based on my reading, DIRFloortime® seemed fairly similar to Son-Rise, so I found a psychologist who was a DIRFloortime® expert to head our home team. He was a world-renowned expert who lectured about this therapy modality far and wide. However, he struggled to engage my son in one-on-one interactions. Of course, the problem was with Anantha, whose understanding of the world was so fragmented and limited!

Other home team members included a speech-language therapist who was good at talking and advocating for funds but little else. There was an occupational therapist with her sensory gym that looked amazing. It was a good half-hour drive each way, but I hoped this would help regulate Anantha's body. It did, temporarily, but by the time his body was regulated, and she felt he could work on some fine motor tasks, it would be time to head home. None of this translated into activities I could do

Chapter 4: Holes

at home with Anantha. Most of our sessions with the speech-language therapist ended with discussions with me since she could not meaningfully work with Anantha in any way. I held on to her because I couldn't find anyone better. She was good at keeping reports organized and team members on point during team meetings. She was also handy when advocating for more therapy hours and funding. Those were her strengths. The bigger unanswered question was, "What were we doing with those hours and funding?" It seems remarkable that not one speech professional at school or home in all those years recommended an Alternative and Augmentative Communication (AAC) device for Anantha. He was a "speaking" child, and AAC was considered appropriate only for non-speaking children. "Those are for severe kids who are cognitively disabled," they responded when I asked about AAC devices. Never mind that Anantha still couldn't tell us if he was hungry or cold. All these years later, Anantha still can't tell us he's hungry by speaking words. At least we have alternate ways of communication to help us now.

Specialized services ended, and a behavioural aide contract started, which meant fewer hours. Some of our professionals left and were replaced by others. Some aides left and were also replaced with new ones. I could go into detail about each professional, but it seems unnecessary. The overriding theme was presumed incompetence. When we first got Anantha's autism diagnosis, I felt a kind of relief that we would receive support from professionals who knew what they were doing. After the ABA debacle, I assumed we had put our trust in the wrong professionals. With the right team, he would soar! It took some time and a few different professionals before I realized that the problem was something different. No one could help us. They didn't know how, and they didn't really care. Also, we didn't have clarity on the help we precisely needed. Everyone showed up for appointments because they had to. No one believed in my child.

Contracts bled into other contracts since they expired every six months. Goals remained unachieved, and we were not allowed to carry them over into a new contract either. We had to develop an entirely new set of goals every six months. It was absurd to keep thinking of new goals to be eligible for support. One of the few exceptions was the occupational therapist. We had switched to an occupational therapist who came to our house and helped with whatever things we had in the home. She had expertise in sensory issues, and her visits were calming to Anantha. She also taught us strategies to help with Anantha's body regulation at school and home. At one point, we let go of all other therapies except the occupational therapist.

After finishing kindergarten in a specialized private setting, Anantha moved on to the public school system to attend a specialized autism program, which meant he would get extra support within a regular classroom. I remember going with him to visit the school and the teachers. The teachers seemed very lovely. I was nervous that it would be hard for Anantha to cope and follow instructions in a crowded classroom. And what would happen when Anantha acted up? Would he be kicked out?

Chapter 4: Holes

That's what trauma does to a person. We are constantly on high alert. We constantly wait for the other shoe to drop. We are scared to trust, let go and hope for the best. These were late lessons for my husband and me and, unfortunately, part of Anantha's life from the beginning. The next few years were probably some of the better ones in Anantha's educational life. Although there were hiccups, he was well-supported in the public-school classroom. His education assistants were very loving and kind. Even though he didn't have a reliable way of showing what he knew, he was in a typical classroom, absorbing all the richness of instruction. He woke up at six o'clock every morning, bright-eyed and eager to go to school. He took the bus to and from school and seemed happy.

Robert

A TYPICAL DAY FOR ANANTHA IN GRADE SEVEN

Anantha's wish to be included in a typical school setting with like-minded peers is a request most children never have to advocate for. By his own account, Anantha knows that being autistic impacts how he participates in learning and school. For example, being in school for long periods or answering questions on the spot can be difficult and stressful. The thing is, Anantha also knows that he *can* learn; it's *how* he participates in learning that is different from other students. To highlight the difference between viewing students as capable based on their ability to conform versus adapting the learning environment to meet the needs and abilities of students, I describe a typical school day for Anantha when he was in grade seven.

To begin each day, I checked in with the teacher before Anantha's arrival. The teacher and I discussed the lesson and possible modifications so that Anantha could participate and achieve the expected learning outcomes. Once Anantha arrived at school, I greeted him at the front doors and quickly connected with Diwakar (Anantha's dad) to learn about any updates, including how Anantha slept, his morning routine, and other pertinent information.

Chapter 4: Holes

Immediately following the routine of Anantha's school entry, he and I walked to the sensory room, where he usually removed his coat and lay on the bean bag for about five minutes. Typically, Anantha requested that the lights are turned off, and the sensory lights (bubble tube, glow-in-the-dark lights) be turned on. Anantha would pull a weighted blanket over himself and wanted the room to be predictably quiet. After settling in, I would ask Anantha how he felt as an initial check-in following the transition into the school building.

Together we made a daily schedule to plan for Anantha's time in school, which ranged from thirty minutes to two hours. The essential components of Anantha's daily program included flexible time in the sensory room, explicitly stated learning goals, movement breaks, predictable peer interactions, and a home-time routine. Anantha learned to trust that the plan we created each day would flex as he needed. Without question, Anantha had the option to move between school spaces as he required and did not need to ask the classroom teacher permission to leave. Anantha also chose to focus on schoolwork in class (usually his preference), or he could work on learning tasks with a small group of peers or me in a breakout space or the sensory room. When in class, Anantha always had access to his communication device where pre-programmed phrases, including "I need a break," "I need a walk," "I need space," and "I need help." Having instant access to a few phrases reduced the pressure on Anantha to use a letter board in moments when he needed to communicate quickly. Occasionally we used a visual timer if Anantha had a goal for the length of time he wanted to remain in class. If I noticed Anantha appeared agitated (louder vocalizations, increased movements), I would offer him a break or ask if he wanted to remain in class. An exciting area of growth for Anantha is that schoolwork became regulating for him. When Anantha was both challenged and supported, it helped his brain and body connect, redirecting his energy into learning and being in class. One of the most critical strategies that led to Anantha's success was regularly checking in with him and using his feedback to make minor adjustments to his schedule and school day. Providing Anantha with many opportunities to offer input helped him achieve personal success because it gave him a choice in decisions that were responsive to him at that moment.

Anantha enjoyed listening to teacher lessons, group discussions and student presentations, so it was a common goal that he stayed in class for those activities. Anantha also liked participating in small group discussions in quiet areas of the school. These discussions were most productive when Anantha could formulate his questions ahead of time so that he felt prepared and confident to converse with his peers. Once Anantha's goal for being in school was reached, or if he felt unsettled, he would request to leave school early. With the support of classroom teachers, parents, and the home support team, Anantha continued to work on his learning tasks from home. His teachers used a daily communication log where they communicated with Anantha about assignments and ongoing work expectations and answered any of Anantha's

Chapter 4: Holes

questions. The opportunity for Anantha to stream into school lessons and group activities validated his sense of belonging. It was clear that Anantha's teachers accepted and respected Anantha for who he was and looked for ways for Anantha to flexibly be a part of the classroom community, even when he wasn't physically present.

Chandra

LEGITIMIZING NON-SPEAKING FORMS OF COMMUNICATION

Approximately one-third of autistic people are non or minimally speaking (Kasari et al., 2014; Jaswal et al., 2020). The use of alternative modes of communication can be traced back to sixteenth-century Europeans and First Nations peoples of North America (Wurtzburg & Campbell, 1995). Early Europeans used sign language to communicate with the deaf, and Indigenous people used forms of manual and pictorial language to communicate with tribes who spoke different languages (Wurtzburg & Campbell, 1995). The development of technology-based Augmentative and Alternative Communication (AAC) devices began in the early nineteenth century to support individuals with severe physical disabilities, specifically those with cerebral palsy (Vanerheiden, 2002). Transferring assistive communication principles to the autistic population did not occur until the 1960s, when communication boards were used with children using early methods of ABA (Donvan & Zucker, 2016). The *United Nations Convention on the Rights of Persons with Disabilities* (2018) defines AAC as methods used to

Chapter 4: Holes

facilitate speech and written communication, including sign language, picture symbols, large print, tactile communication, plain language, multimedia, and technologies such as speech-generating devices. For individuals considered intelligible (Bergenmar et al., 2015), the use of generated speech allows non and minimally speaking people to communicate more freely.

Tools such as AAC devices create opportunities for minimally and non-speaking autistic people to communicate feelings, needs, thoughts, and experiences with loved ones, participate in learning, socialize, and live more independent lives. However, it is essential to recognize that ableist structures are embedded in many of our supports for autistic students, including AAC devices. For instance, for some non or minimally speaking autistic persons to enter dialogue using an AAC, they are first expected to conform to implicitly governed non-autistic speaking modes of address (Ellsworth, 1997). Pre-programmed symbols, pictures and vocabularies predominantly reflect society's neurotypical preferences for conversational topics and experiences. For instance, suppose an autistic person wanted to share a unique experience, such as how he "sees" his mother's voice (Higashida, 2016, para 6). Most often, this experience would not be represented in a neurotypically pre-programmed AAC device, or if an autistic person were able to spell out their experience, the legitimacy would be questioned and most likely corrected because of non-autistic dissonance such as "you can't see your mother's voice!".

Consequently, authentic representation and expression of the experience and, by extension, autistic identity become unrecognized or muted. This example shows how deeply embedded ableist structures are, even within our evidence-based practices. While we understand and appreciate that the primary goal of AAC is to facilitate efficient and effective communication (Beukelman & Mirenda, 2005); the use of AAC also has the potential to decontextualize the autistic individual from their authentic experiences and selves (Taylor, 1992). Over time, through repeated mis or non-recognition, communicative biology may be replaced with socially preferred communicative behaviours, essentially denying the authentic self to be viewed as so-called normal (Bergenmar et al., 2015). Additionally, the burden of conforming to typical modes of social communication (Ashby & Causton-Theoharis, 2009) and self-translating experience into textual thoughts (Bergenmar et al., 2015) becomes unevenly placed on the non or minimally speaking autistic person.

When society perpetually echoes beliefs of deficit, inability and fault onto disabled people, the idea of the self as belonging becomes distorted (Taylor, 1992), often leading to masking and internalized oppression (Barnes & Oliver, 2012). Autistic individuals' perceived lack of social competence and repeated rejection of authentic self contribute to higher reports of anxiety and depression compared to the non-autistic population (Cage et al., 2018; Chandrasekhar & Sikich, 2015). In education, the abilities of autistic individuals are measured against standardized cognitive, speech, and motor assessments

Chapter 4: Holes

that are normed on non-autistic ways of being—including thinking, moving, and communicating; consequently, underestimating or overlooking (Zeliadt, 2018) autistic ability and intelligence. To avoid errors in recognizing student ability, educators must consider how formal and informal assessments perpetuate ableist ideas and expectations of neurotypical ability.

CHAPTER 5: LIGHT

Freedom Dance

Tap.
Tap.
A tentative pointer,
Quivering,
Caressing shyly,
The 26 keys to enlightenment.
Each tap,
Radiating skyward,
Showering wisdom,
To brethren.
Choreographing,
A thunderous stomp.
Thud.
Thud.
Thud.
Thud.
Marching to the devils' lair,
Shattering sordid stories,
With resounding resonance.
Thanks, oh seminal finger,
For revealing to me,
The freedom dance.

~Anantha

Anantha

Holes allow light to shine through. My mom was my shining light and a beacon of hope during dark times. She refused to believe the experts, often enduring ridicule from even those close to her. Snide comments from skeptics did not deter her from exposing me to age-appropriate reading, writing, and math. She discovered a communication method that allowed me to express my actual thoughts and feelings by pointing at the alphabet on a letter board. This allowed me to show the world the intact brain trapped within a wretched body.

The real me finally revealed itself to a scarcely believing world. A me that can do well in academics if supported meaningfully. A me that can contribute to society instead of being a burden. A me that can enrich the diversity of voices in our world. A me that will fight to make sure no other non-speaking autistic person suffers the indignities so callously inflicted on me.

I am still an anxious, angry, and aggressive mess. My autism is creating many obstacles for me to function in a society constructed with a bias against neurodiversity. Mere symbolic acceptance and awareness aren't enough. A revolution is a need of the hour—a new civil rights movement to end the discrimination against neuro-divergence.

I digress. So, what is my manual?

Janani

STRANGE COINCIDENCES

In 2014 I started reading a blog called Emma's Hope Book. It was an incredibly well-written blog and very nuanced. I don't remember what led me to it, but I was hooked because Emma sounded exactly like Anantha. She spoke in scripted sentences and seemingly random phrases. If you based your opinion of her understanding on her spoken words, it would seem that she understood little. However, her mother had taken her to Texas to meet Soma Mukhopadhyay, who helped Emma communicate her thoughts. The method Soma used was called the Rapid Prompting Method (RPM). I wondered, "Could this be helpful for Anantha too? Did he understand much more than we believed?" In March 2014, I contacted HALO, the non-profit agency where Soma worked and tried to enroll in a workshop. I was told that all spots were full for spring and summer, but perhaps we could register in the fall instead.

Sometimes strange coincidences happen. I had hired a play therapist trained in Son-Rise as an additional aide to play with Anantha once a week. She brought up the topic of RPM on her own, having heard about it from a friend in the province of British Columbia. She didn't know how to do it, and neither did I, but we attempted a session to imitate what we'd learned in some online videos. We didn't have much success, and she moved away from Calgary shortly after. Then another mom in Calgary posted on Facebook asking if anyone had tried RPM for their child. She planned to call an RPM provider trained under Soma to come to Calgary to provide a workshop. I connected with her and offered to help in any way possible. It would be considerably cheaper to partner with someone than go to Texas.

We managed to get six interested families, and we were going to split the costs of the workshop amongst ourselves. The provider would work with our children, and we would receive videos of the sessions to use as a reference for our home programs. The workshop happened over three days in March 2015. Jackie Dorshorst, the RPM provider, had travelled from Wisconsin to do the workshop. The participants ranged from young kids to adults in their 20s. She would work with each individual one-on-one in a small room, and a live feed of the session would be broadcast to all the other families and participants waiting in another room. The day before the workshop, I was an anxious wreck!

"Would my son respond to the new method? Have I subjected him to some new torture because of my expectations?" Jackie started the session by sitting beside Anantha and telling him the sky was "blue." Then she asked if she had said the sky was "blue" or "yellow," writing each colour down on individual pieces of paper.

Chapter 5: Light

Anantha pointed to "blue." She then talked about how we see clouds in the sky. Jackie then asked Anantha to spell "white" by showing him a large stencil with letters. He spelled the word out, to my surprise, with a bit of physical prompting. Jackie was talking to him as if he understood everything, and he was responding as if he did understand everything that was being said. Mind-blowing!

I spent most of those three days in a very emotional state, feeling weepy and celebratory. It was a life-changing, paradigm-shifting weekend. Every single one of the autistic participants had responded to Jackie's instruction. Her lessons ranged from simple topics like rain for younger children to more mature topics like Gandhi and non-violence for older individuals. She had a calm, engaging manner and an attitude that radiated belief in a person's ability to understand and be taught the new communication method.

I had thought others were underestimating my son, but I had not realized how much I was guilty of it myself. I had talked down to him, not sure if he understood. I hadn't read age-appropriate books to him or thought he could learn without mind-numbing repetition. "If he is so smart, why is he not talking? Why is he not typing?" were questions we asked ourselves. In fact, Anantha understood everything but had trouble getting his mouth to reply with the correct words. Jackie explained that speaking was complicated and took more muscle control than pointing fingers. Pointing with fingers had to be learned slowly since the body instinctively reverted to familiar movement and speech patterns, which explained Anantha's verbal stims and loops! Although Jackie provided clear explanations for some autistic people's inability to speak or independently type, the new information didn't sink in until I read more blogs and the personal experiences of autistic people. It has taken us years to understand the complexity of Anantha's struggles.

It was one thing for Jackie to help Anantha spell words. It was quite another for me to attempt it at home. Although Jackie had given us sample lesson plans and even completed a session where we did the teaching, and she observed, RPM seemed incredibly daunting. I would attempt lessons for a week and then give them up for a short while. The longer the gap, the more daunting it got. Preparing content was the easy part. Delivering RPM lessons and remaining calm, even if Anantha got dysregulated, was difficult for me. I was inclined to lose my calm, sometimes just as quickly as Anantha. Our sessions would end with both of us yelling in frustration and close to tears. You might wonder why Anantha needs someone to help him communicate using a letter board. The person who supports Anantha type also helps to regulate Anantha so that he can communicate through typing. This can be viewed as a form of co-regulation and communication support. The communication partner and Anantha must establish trust and comfort to effectively co-regulate. It is like a dance that flows between dance partners as they become more familiar with one another.

Chapter 5: Light

NAVIGATING PUBLIC EDUCATION, SPECIAL EDUCATION, HOME SCHOOL, AND PRIVATE SCHOOL

GRADE THREE: PUBLIC EDUCATION

Meanwhile, things were getting harder for Anantha in 2016 when he attended a specialized class for autistic students in a public school. He needed one-on-one support full-time, something the school found hard to provide, especially with funding cuts. Questions began to be asked about how much Anantha understood and if he belonged in the program. A specialized placement within the public school began to be marketed to me as a better fit for Anantha. It would provide a calmer environment, and he would receive more support. The school completed a psych-ed assessment for Anantha, which was a disaster without any support. Anantha picked up on all the stress and, as a result, became fraught with anxiety himself, struggling with dysregulation at school and home. I tried sharing videos of his RPM sessions with the school team. I even presented copies of the book *Ido in Autismland* to his teacher. I couldn't win this fight. The writing was on the wall. He would be in a special education placement in a public school for grade four. Everyone urged us to give it a try. Maybe it wouldn't be so bad. Perhaps the extra support would help Anantha's nervous system calm down and pave the way to learning. Maybe pigs would fly!

GRADE FOUR: SPECIAL EDUCATION

We gave the specialized classroom a try for three months in 2017, during which time I volunteered at different times of the day to try and understand the routines. Yes, there was more staff, but the expectations were so much lower. My daughter was four years old and learning more than Anantha in grade four. At home, Anantha stopped wanting to work with me, and he seemed to have given up completely. I knew that homeschooling was our best option at that point. However, I still didn't feel confident enough to support him.

Consequently, I decided to make the trip to Texas to see Soma and attend the four-day parent training on RPM. It was a fantastic time; I made many new friends and learned new things! I came home bubbling with ideas and activities to implement. We had Megan, a young and enthusiastic aide, start working with Anantha. She was very interested in RPM and willing to learn about it. We decided to pull Anantha from his special education class and homeschool him to focus on developing communication.

GRADES FOUR AND FIVE: HOME SCHOOL

Between us, we launched into a full-time home school program for the remainder of Anantha's grade four year and all of grade five. Megan took Anantha to homeschool classes organized by a group. I would prepare lessons about different topics like ocean ecosystems and garbage collection for Megan to teach Anantha at home. In 2018,

Chapter 5: Light

I organized a workshop with Soma Mukhopadhyay in Calgary. It went very well, inspiring Megan to take up the method with more students. She went to Texas to train and, in a few months and started her practice here in Calgary. She now works with several autistic individuals and their families, changing their lives through communication and education. We lucked out and found a psychologist who has been helpful as a counsellor, a speech-language therapist who helped us with AAC trials, and an occupational therapist and physiotherapist who helped with Anantha's body regulation. Despite all our efforts, Anantha did not like being homeschooled. He viewed it as a punishment and wanted nothing more than to be back in a typical classroom among kids his age. He became increasingly resistant to working with us, especially me. He told us he wanted to be back in school full-time.

GRADE SIX: SPECIAL EDUCATION IN A PRIVATE SCHOOL

Although, in theory, the very word inclusion indicates everyone, I knew one of the biggest roadblocks to Anantha attending a typical classroom was his previous psychoeducational assessment completed when Anantha was in grade three. Therefore, we went to a private psychologist to request a modified assessment that would allow the presence of a letterboard and a communication partner. The psychologist was initially reluctant but agreed after watching Anantha spell and was convinced of his independence in communication. Anantha tested at an average level for reading comprehension, listening comprehension, numerical operations, math problem solving and spelling and writing skills. His verbal comprehension was very high, in the 98th percentile! His visual-spatial skills and working memory were on the lower side, likely affected by his poor fine motor and visual-motor abilities. I have since come to understand that intelligence scores are problematic and should not be used as gatekeeping measures that permit or restrict access to education. However, at the time, I was willing to do whatever it took to ensure that a school board would take Anantha seriously. The cognitive assessment was more of a tool for school placement than for us to understand Anantha better.

Armed with this new assessment, we approached the public-school board and some of Calgary's private schools. Calling around and making inquiries, I understood that most private schools that provided a general education were inherently biased at the very mention of autism. Some of them hung up or sweetly suggested the names of some autism-specific schools. The private schools specifically for kids with disabilities were not quite the right match either. One of them was very ABA-based and not even on our radar. Another took only "high-functioning" kids since they focused on academics and were not set up to support other types of learners. Everywhere there was a hierarchy, and my son, with his severe support needs, ranked at the very bottom. He was not deemed worthy of a typical education, not even spending a few minutes in a general education classroom.

Chapter 5: Light

In 2019, after a brief failed attempt at our neighbourhood school, we enrolled Anantha in one of the city's special education schools that focused on academic programming. This new school agreed to provide an education assistant specifically to support Anantha. In return, we would have to pay almost twice the fees compared to the other parents. We were desperate for this educational placement to work, so we borrowed from our line of credit to finance the tuition. Without getting into too many specifics, I will tell you that it wasn't what we had hoped for. The school appeared better in theory when we toured the campus. Then COVID-19 happened, and everything shifted online. It was a vast unsustainable drain of resources for a non-return. Yet, we didn't have any other option for the upcoming 2020-21 academic year, which was to be Anantha's grade seven-year.

INCLUSIVE EDUCATION

Through a stroke of luck, Anantha was accepted through a lottery process to the Science School for grade seven in the public school system. Initially, we had several meetings with numerous people to advocate for support. Everyone was incredibly supportive of his learning profile and needs, and we have had a positive experience overall! However, his severe sensory and emotional dysregulation means he cannot attend school for more than a few minutes on some days. This means that his work is sent home to be completed when he is able. How is this different from homeschooling, you might ask? He still belongs to a class and has classmates; this sense of belonging has been critical to Anantha's emotional well-being. There is also the hope that he will be able to stay longer and participate in more in-class activities on his better days.

For the better part of Anantha's grade seven-year in 2020, my husband became the primary communication partner for Anantha. My husband is better regulated than I am, which I think is incredibly important for the success of a communication partner. Since my husband has become Anantha's primary communication partner at home, Anantha's creative writing has blossomed. Anantha has had several of his poems and stories published online.

We don't know what the future holds, especially in terms of education for Anantha, but we are now taking it one day at a time and hoping for positive outcomes.

Robert

KINDNESS AND COMPASSION

I am drawn to the humanness of Anantha's life story and his fierce desire to receive an education. When I think about the concept of humanness in education, I am reminded of the powerful impact Anantha's peers have on his sense of school belonging.

Anantha has often shared that feeling and being included at school has positively impacted his mental health. I believe Anantha's self-observation of the improvements to his mental health is primarily due to the efforts and commitment made by school leaders and teachers to create a school-wide culture of acceptance and belonging. One way Anantha's school exhibits a culture of inclusion is how the student body shows kindness and compassion towards Anantha. For example, there was an instance at the start of Anantha's grade seven school year when Anantha and I worked together to prepare a personal bio to present to Anantha's classmates and teacher. Anantha shared information on his favourite foods, movies, and books, the places he wished to travel to, and the superpowers he wanted to try. Anantha's classmates were very intrigued, and I could tell they were interested in getting to know Anantha better. It struck me that Anantha's classmates saw the similarities between themselves and Anantha, not just the differences. The only noticeable distinction between Anantha and his peers was that he used an iPad to communicate, and his body moved differently to regulate or show emotion.

As a whole class, we talked about Anantha's stims, what they look like (including licking his fingers or vocalizations), and what they meant. Part of our discussion included asking Anantha's classmates to share what they did to help them feel calm if they felt anxious or had trouble focusing. Anantha's classmates quickly shared several examples, including "go grab some water," "twirl my pencil," "tap my leg on the ground," "play with my hair," "bite my nails," and "listen to music." One student summarized our discussion with the comment, "So I guess you could say that all these things are ways we try and stay focused; it is just different for everyone?" During our discussion, the kindness, compassion, and understanding that Anantha's peers displayed showed me that students are often more accepting than we give them credit for.

Later in the school year, Anantha's conversation with his peers during a social studies lesson resonated with me. It highlighted how even in the smallest of actions, I could see how attuned, kind, and supportive Anantha's peers were to him. A few students spoke with Anantha about inclusion and how inclusive and exclusionary practices have evolved. One of his peers abruptly turned to me and said, "Hey, Mr. C, when can Anantha stay long enough to

Chapter 5: Light

have lunch with us? We play lots of cool games sometimes. I think he might like to play. He should be included".

There would be times when I was in class with Anantha when I found my anxiety increasing because I wondered and worried about Anantha's classmate's feelings and thoughts on Anantha. I would continually think several steps ahead to try and ensure all possibilities were considered so that Anantha did not feel judged by his classmates and that Anantha felt like he belonged. For example, there were several times when I held my breath when I noticed Anantha's anxiety increasing if a peer asked him a question. I wasn't sure if Anantha was ready to answer or if Anantha would start talking loudly about trains, babysitters, or random words strung together that did not appear to make sense. At first, I thought Anantha's classmates would respond by whispering or making inappropriate or insensitive comments. Anantha and his dignity were always so important to me. I wanted to protect him as much as possible during moments when his brain and body did not appear in sync. I was constantly reminded that Anantha's classmates cared immensely. There were no sideways looks or inappropriate comments. However, I know Anantha's classmates were curious, which is a normal response and should be expected and responded to. Because Anantha's teachers highly respected Anantha, so did his peers. For example, a peer approached Anantha after a lesson ended by asking him what he thought about the video they watched in class. Anantha began to make loud vocalizations and appeared uncomfortable. The student graciously responded to Anantha, "It's okay,

Anantha; maybe I can email you my question instead." I am constantly in awe of Anantha's peers at school, their genuine kindness, compassion, and respect for Anantha, and how willing and able they are to make sure Anantha continually feels like an essential member of the school community.

Chandra

IS INCLUSIVE POLICY AND PRACTICE WORKING?

There are several international laws and policies that provide countries with definitions and frameworks for inclusive education. The United Nations Education, Scientific and Cultural Organization (UNESCO) published a global education report that evaluates over 160 countries' commitments to achieving six goals to improve learning opportunities for children, youth, and adults (Global Education Monitoring Report, 2020). However, researchers defend that "no country has yet succeeded in constructing a school system that lives up to the ideals and intentions of inclusion" (Haug, 2017, p.206). This shortcoming appears to result from breakdowns between inclusive education ideas and the realities of students and schools. Leaders, teachers, and parents philosophically agree with the concept of equal educational rights for students with disabilities. However, they are uncertain about how best to create systems and environments that support the unique needs of students with diverse abilities across the grades (Haug, 2017; Messiou, 2019; Mitchell & Sutherland, 2020).

While viewing education as an integrated whole between students' heads and hearts is improving, too commonly, seeking the viewpoints from the disabled community on how best to enact this is undervalued or is a tokenistic add-on. Self-advocacy groups and social justice movements continue to carry the weight of reforming exclusionary practices, including "nothing about us, without us" (Chown et al., 2017). Yet educators are often unaware that micro-exclusions continue to exist within anti-oppressive school initiatives, including less than adequate representation of students with disabilities within anti-racism, anti-bullying, or LGBTQIA2S+ initiatives.

AUTISTIC STUDENTS AND THEIR SCHOOL EXPERIENCES

As the prevalence of autism has increased, so has autism-related research; however, like jurisdictional practices, most research reflects researcher, medical, educator, and parent perspectives (DePape & Lindsay, 2016). Very little research centres exclusively on autistic students' perspectives and self-reported school experiences (Lebenhagen, 2022; Woodfield & Ashby, 2016). For example, since 2000, approximately 23 studies have been published that sought the self-reported experiences of autistic students, and since 2016, only three studies and three meta-syntheses have been published. This lack of literature reflects ableist research practices and views on non-normative ability, contributing to outdated and ineffective teaching practices to support autistic students in education.

Chapter 5: Light

Based on currently available research, autistic students identify eight main areas as either positively or negatively contributing to their overall school experiences, which include a) diagnostic labelling, b) sensory issues, c) stigmatizing supports, d) boredom, e) curriculum workload f) peer relationships, g) transitions and routines, and h) teacher characteristics (Danker et al., 2016; DePape & Lindsay, 2016; Dillon et al., 2016; Lebenhagen, 2022; Woodfiled & Ashby, 2016).

Throughout these chapters, Anantha and Janani shared personal stories affirming research on autistic students' reported school experiences. Medical, educational, and social belief systems and practices that aim to reshape the autistic person into "normal," "typical," "standard," and "averages" have severe and long-lasting harmful effects on autistic people and their families. In the following chapter, Anantha, Janani, Robert, and I offer practical suggestions and reflective questions to create provocations for policymakers, jurisdictional leaders, and educators to consider ways to improve the inclusive education experiences and well-being of neurodivergent students.

CHAPTER 6: MANUAL

Magic Mirror

Mirror mirror on the wall.
Is my baby the best of them all?
Mum mum, not at all.
The atypical quirks need to fall.
Smother him in therapy that is a squall.
To mould him normal overall.
Really wise experts wait for your call.

Mirror mirror on the wall.
I went out and called them all.
My baby took the darkest fall.
The smile is gone from my doll.
Rewards have made him an
anxious troll.
Should he go through this grizzly maul?

Mum mum, stand firm and tall.
Your baby is human not at all.
Enduring conversion is his call.
A joyful childhood you must stall.

Mirror mirror on the wall.
Stop your rhymes and take your pall.
My darling will stim with gall.
His flapping doesn't make him small.
Soar he will to heaven's thrall.
Mirror mirror on the wall.
Shatter you I will with a cannonball.
Lest you blind another eyeball.

~Anantha

Anantha

MY TOP THREE WISHES

MY USER MANUAL IS DECEPTIVELY EASY.

1. Accept my autism. I learn differently. I have unique strengths and challenges, just like others. Adapt my education instead of extinguishing my autism.
2. Presume competence. I am capable of learning age-appropriate content. Non-speaking doesn't mean non-thinking. Don't judge a book by its cover. Treat me with the same respect you would afford to a neurotypical.
3. Show me love and kindness. This gives me the incredible strength to rise above my wretched autistic body.

JANANI

MY ADVICE FOR PARENTS OF AUTISTIC CHILDREN

If you've made it this far, you would have noticed that regret is heavily interwoven in my story. There are so many things I wish I had done differently for my son. In 2015 my daughter was diagnosed with autism as well. Partly due to the lessons learned from our experiences with parenting Anantha, we chose differently for my daughter. From the beginning, her educational placement has been in an inclusive classroom with support. We chose a Montessori preschool over a regular preschool since it tended to be a quieter environment better suited to her learning needs. She flourished and thrived in that placement. We steered clear of ABA and examined what support she needed at every stage. I hope my narrative will help other parents explore options and choose better for their children.

In no particular order, I have listed below some ideas that I invite other parents to consider when choosing support for their children.

Rethink the Objectives of Therapy: There is enough evidence to suggest that early childhood trauma, particularly in the first five years of life, can have long-lasting effects on personality and regulation. No one would ever say their therapy objective is to cause trauma, and we would never even look at it that way. Aren't we just trying to help our children play better, socialize better, fit in, and make friends? Consider what this entails, however. Are we saying that the ways our children naturally play, communicate, and socialize are wrong? Are we unwittingly sending a message that our children are not enough, just the way they are? How does this impact their self-image and self-esteem? We love them with all our hearts; of course, they are enough. However, this may not be the message they receive when forced to undergo hours of intervention and therapy.

Instead of buying into the frenzied treatments and interventions, pause and consider what your child truly needs. First and foremost, it would help your child feel more comfortable in their body. This could mean enlisting the help of an occupational therapist for sensory strategies and activities that help them cope with their unique sensory system. While sensory overload is common among many autistic people, not everyone responds to sensory stimuli similarly. Physiotherapy can be beneficial as well. Many non-speaking autistic people struggle with motor planning and coordination, and a physiotherapist can provide some valuable strategies to help autistic people with some of these issues.

Equally critical is communication. Introduce alternative methods of communication, such as AAC, as soon as possible, especially if your child is non-speaking or not fluently speaking. Waiting for spoken language and

Chapter 6: Manual

prioritizing this over any other communication form is a huge disservice to your child. Wanting to communicate but being unable to do so can be incredibly frustrating in ways we don't understand because we take speech for granted. There is a myth that introducing AAC will make the child too reliant on it as a communication method, and they won't even try to speak with their mouth. This is not true and problematic in assuming that spoken words are somehow superior. Working on mouth speech can be a separate parallel goal, alongside exploring alternate communication methods.

Listen to Autistic Voices: We are fortunate to live in a time when many autistic self-advocates share their perspectives and experiences on blogs, websites, and social media groups. When I first came across a blog written by an autistic person, I told my husband, "If our son could write like this online, I would consider him cured." I had made the common ableist assumption that having high support needs equated to being cognitively disabled. I assumed that the people who wrote fluently online had no support needs and lived independent lives. At times, I felt annoyed that these people would dare speak on behalf of someone who was so not exactly like them. Now I know better. Not only because my son writes beautifully, but he also has areas of intense struggle. Over the past several years, I've joined a lot of autistic-led spaces on Facebook, I follow autistic advocates on Twitter, and I read publications like Neuroclastic, which provide a wealth of information exclusively from autistic people. I mostly read and listen. Not everything discussed applies to me, and

I take what is relevant. I continue to learn every single day. However, this does require setting aside your ego as a parent and not taking critiques and opposing information personally. Remember that autistic self-advocates are volunteering their time and energy, which doesn't come easy, to try and smooth the way for future generations. Getting offended at the tone or even the content is counterproductive.

Don't Be Apologetic About Advocating: This is an area I am still working on. I have been taught from my childhood to keep my head down and not make a fuss. This is both cultural in origin and because I am a woman. Becoming a parent to autistic kids has been a lesson in the opposite. "The squeaky wheel gets the grease" has been said to me many times by well-meaning people. It is, unfortunately, true. Our children need us to advocate for them. This also helps our children understand that their needs matter, that they matter. In time, advocacy is something that they will have to be responsible for themselves.

Look Into Your Neurodivergence: Apples don't fall far from the tree. I was diagnosed with ADHD (Inattentive) last year, and it explains a lot about everything! A diagnosis has helped me understand why I struggle to do certain things and excel at others. My neurodivergence helped me avoid constantly comparing myself to other parents, looking for all the ways I fall short. My diagnosis has allowed me to ask for help in places I struggle. This perspective change, in turn, has touched other parts of my life, like parenting. It has helped me understand my kids' challenges and be a better advocate.

I could add more to this list, but many things depend on individual circumstances. I hope the above list helps parents of newly diagnosed autistic children avoid making some of my mistakes.

Robert

TIPS FOR TEACHERS

Knowing that the makeup of today's classrooms is increasingly diverse, teaching students with complex learning, communication, and sensory presentations may feel daunting to many teachers. As an educator, I tell you that having neurodiverse students in your class is a gift to you and the other students. Inclusion begins with a mindset, and I have seen how successful inclusion can be for students and teachers when teams look for opportunities rather than barriers. Based on my experiences as a classroom teacher and walking alongside colleagues in many different schools, I share the following practical, strength-based strategies to support the inclusion of autistic students.

In-School Champion: An essential first step to supporting meaningful inclusion for autistic students is identifying an in-school champion. This point-person is a consistent conduit for sharing information between teachers, administration, support personnel, parents, and students. Having an in-school champion forms the basis for developing solid student-teacher relationships, which is key to identifying responsive and practical strategies to support students. For Anantha, having a point person (myself) allowed our shared goals to be clearly identified and consistently reviewed in strategic and strength-based ways. As an in-school champion, I shared my knowledge, modelled inclusive thinking and problem-solving, and built trust with my colleagues. I also co-explored ways Anantha's non-speaking voice could be included in decision-making about academic learning, peer relationships, and his sensory needs.

Co-Advocacy and Self-Advocacy: Through the advocacy and support from an in-school champion, the student's voice is included in all decision-making about schedules, access to sensory and learning spaces, engagement in curriculum, assessment, and communication with teachers and peers. Co-advocacy helps build understanding, trust, and respect between team members and autistic students. As Anantha shared, "non-speaking does not mean non-thinking." Therefore, to support self-advocacy, consider ways you include student voices that do not rely on speaking forms of communication.

Rethink Time and Space to Build Inclusive Communities: Using time and space is one of the most critical factors in students' overall feelings of academic success, belonging, and safety. When teachers evaluate the effectiveness of specific supports and strategies, time and space considerations are helpful. Often, it is not the strategy that is ineffective; instead, the space and time in which the strategy is used is the problem. When scheduling a student's timetable, the helpful question is, "How can different school spaces be used to make learning more accessible to students with disabilities?"

Kindness and Compassion: Be empathetic towards different types of human experience. Seek to understand student differences instead of viewing representations of student ability from a singular, neurotypical perspective. When we seek to understand, we learn to be vulnerable, which opens space for our learning and growth as humans and teachers. Take time to learn about the autistic student's story by asking questions. What works, and what doesn't? What are their passions? What makes them feel anxious and scared? What are their goals and dreams? Find ways for autistic students to share their stories, from their point of view, in personally meaningful ways, including non-speaking forms. With kindness and compassion, listen to students' stories by hearing, seeing, and attuning.

Chandra

CREATING INCLUSIVE SCHOOL CULTURES

Combining first-hand perspectives with current research offers educational leaders, teachers, and parents exciting and progressive opportunities to reflect on and reform their beliefs. However, ideas are not enough. While new truths from neurodivergent students expand our viewpoints, educators must also consider how this new knowledge is mobilized within schools and school jurisdictions. To truly build inclusive school cultures for the 21st century, perspectives from the disabled student community must be integrated into the very core of diversity, equity, inclusion, and access initiatives. Tokenistic add-ons do not lead to meaningful or sustainable change, nor does it replace deeply entrenched ableist beliefs and processes.

Below I offer reflective questions for jurisdictional leaders, school administrators, and teachers to consider as they work toward removing barriers and improving access to meaningful inclusion for students.

1. Do policies and processes require students to provide medical documentation to be eligible for support and accommodations?

2. Do jurisdictional practices unduly emphasize remediation, subsequently implying that students are responsible for overcoming barriers to inclusion?
3. In what ways are the perspectives of students with disabilities sought to inform inclusive practices and initiatives?
4. What evidence is collected to understand if schools are welcoming, caring, and safe places for students with disabilities?
5. In what ways do school jurisdiction proactively partner with parents of disabled students?
6. How are the intersectional identities of disabled students (race, ethnicity, sexuality, and gender) represented in school initiatives, including anti-bullying and LGBTQIA2s+?
7. What job-embedded coaching and mentorship opportunities are available to teachers and support staff to increase their understanding, skill, and confidence in teaching students with disabilities?
8. How is perception data from disabled and non-disabled students, teachers, parents, and external stakeholders integrated to evaluate and inform inclusive policy and practices?
9. How are diversity and equity considered in the distribution of resources to support students with disabilities in inclusion?
10. What school-wide actions demonstrate to the student population that inclusion is an individual participatory experience?

Chapter 6: Manual

The following simple Venn diagram summarizes our collective beliefs on the core elements educators should pay attention to as they seek ways to include autistic students more ethically, equitably, and meaningfully in school. First, accept autistic students as they are. Second, presume competence and ability instead of believing differences equates with deficits. Third, seek to meaningfully include the voice of autistic students in personally relevant decisions, including the ordinary events of day-to-day school life. Fourth, show kindness, compassion, and patience to those who, by no choice of their own, experience the world differently.

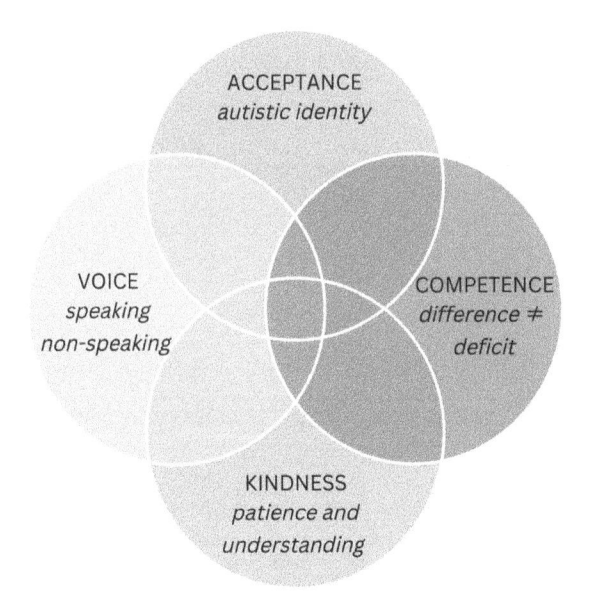

ACCEPTANCE
autistic identity

VOICE
*speaking
non-speaking*

COMPETENCE
*difference ≠
deficit*

KINDNESS
*patience and
understanding*

CHAPTER 7: FINAL REFLECTIONS

The Last Gate

Slam!
A slap on the soul.
Slam!
A sentence of solitude.
Slam!
A lash for not conforming.
Slam!
A scar from entrenched bigotry.
Door.
After dark door.
Blocking the spirit.
Nails to the coffin of dreams.
Door.
After dark door.
Save.
The last golden gate.
Unhinged by openness.
Showering radiant compassion.
From kindred Celeste's.
Stars aligned in a cosmic mission.
To open portals.
From the deathly stench
of segregation.
To the exalted senses of inclusion.

~Anantha

LOOKING BACK, LOOKING FORWARD

SPRING 2022

We tell stories to help us make sense of events, share knowledge, construct our identities, and connect with others. We hope that by listening to our stories, your ideas about autism, ability, disability, and inclusion have changed and that you feel encouraged to seek new ways to include autistic people, and others with disabilities, more ethically and equitably in all aspects of education and community. Through Anantha's voice, we learned that a significant issue impacting the lives of autistic people is the enaction of theories developed by non-autistic people on what it means to receive a meaningful education as an autistic person. We also learned that honouring autistic people's representations of voice is the most practical and principled way we can disrupt ableist assumptions and practices that overshadow first-person perspectives.

It has been over a year since Anantha, Janani, Diwakar, Robert, and I embarked on our journey of connecting, sharing, learning, and writing together. We have reflected and grown since writing the first chapter together. As we conclude our time together, we share parting reflections based on current knowledge, space, time, and politics.

Anantha

NOW THAT I AM IN GRADE 8

> *"What are your thoughts on the Ukraine-Russia war?"*
> *"How in your mind should a non-disabled person address a disabled person?"*
> *"With a hypotenuse of 13 m, what is the largest area isosceles right triangle one can build?"*

These questions greet me when I open my daily communication journal. The teachers treat me the same as my classmates, and I am expected to do the same assignments and participate in group projects. Yet, they do treat me differently, in a good way. I am provided with a communication partner who supports me one-on-one at school. He adapts his support to match my strengths and does not impose outdated and dangerous behaviour therapy on me. Work is adapted so that I can work on them at my pace and from my destination of choice. I am allowed to retreat into a sensory room when the classroom becomes too overwhelming.

I spend only half a day at school. However, my teachers never forget to include me while I am gone. My presentations are played with text-to-speech to the class, and I am allowed to video conference into class discussions. I was asked to write a poem for Remembrance Day, and the poem was recited at the school assembly by my classmate. The school principal wrote a personal note about how proud she was of me. My silence does not deter anyone from including me.

I do have a team of experts to support me. However, for the first time, my voice and vision are respected. I vet every single decision. For example, my time at school gradually increased based on continuous feedback from me, and this helped me adapt much better to sensory overload. The Individualized Program Plan (IPP) lists me as the first member of my core support team!

The halls of my school are filled with the sweet fragrance of presuming competence. I dearly hope to breathe this air wherever my academic journey takes me.

JANANI

BELIEVING IN INCLUSION

It's been a year and a half since we embarked on this inclusion journey. A journey made stranger by Covid-19 and all that it entailed. I wonder if that helped us in some ways since learning online has become more common. I have been a bit of an observer for this part of my son's life. There are many reasons for this, which I will not get into. Fortunately for us, my husband could step into the role of Anantha's primary communication partner and support person. This means he has had to schedule his work and meetings around Anantha's school schedule and assignments. He has consciously prioritized Anantha's education. I realize this is a privilege for our family. Not everyone has a job with the flexibility to do these things. This will not be an option for my husband in a few months. What happens, then? That's a question with no easy answers. I hope that I will be able to get back to working with Anantha in some capacity.

For us, inclusion has been a journey of advocacy and sheer luck. We were lucky to have the support and knowledge of people like Robert and Chandra, who have helped the school view Anantha differently and structure his support accordingly. We were lucky that he had such excellent teachers who understood the kind of learner Anantha is. Anantha's teachers consistently adjust the schoolwork expected from him, so he is challenged but not fatigued. They also ensure Anantha gets a chance to participate in book clubs and group projects. Not everyone will run into this kind of luck when advocating for their child, and we certainly didn't for years. We kept trying because Anantha wanted an age-appropriate education in a setting with his peers.

I recently spoke at a parent panel regarding my son's school experience in an inclusive classroom with support. The de facto assumption from other parents and people in the advocacy organization was that my son needed minimal help and was well-regulated. Nothing could be further from the truth. If my son, who requires significant support, can be meaningfully supported, and included in school, I'll wager your child can be supported too. It begins with the belief that your child is worthy of being supported in an inclusive classroom. The idea is that they are worthy of an education and capable of learning great and complicated things. The nuts and bolts of it can be worked out later.

Robert

CHAMPIONING INCLUSION

I have learned that although we, as teachers, have good intentions, ableism is entrenched in many of our school processes and teaching practices. Mostly, we lack authentic student input, especially if a student is non-speaking or "behavioural." My time in schools has left me knowing, for a fact, that in most instances, peers are accepting and often more inclusive in their actions and friendships than adults. Students understand the ever-changing, diverse makeup of the society around them and seek to build upon their friendships at school. In many ways, the adults are stuck and need to reconsider their views. When we remind ourselves that solutions are found within students' voices, we are better positioned to see opportunities and become more effective and honourable in our practice.

Our collective mindsets, which viewed Anantha and his parents as equal partners, helped us create a supportive framework to help Anantha reach his academic and social goals in flexible ways that respected his unique abilities and support needs. This framework can be applied to any student to help them achieve personal success in inclusion. Working alongside Anantha, his parents, and the school team, has been an exceptional experience and has caused me to reflect deeply on my practice and beliefs on inclusion and acceptance. I strongly encourage my fellow educators to seek new ways to understand their students' personal stories and create spaces where students can safely share their hopes and wishes for the future. My hope for educators reading our stories is that they see themselves in the celebrations and the challenges and recognize that the best inclusive strategies do not come in pre-packaged bundles. Instead, identifying the most effective and responsive strategy is found in students' voices, perspectives, and actions.

Anantha taught me that every student deserves the right to education alongside their peers. Anantha reminded me that meaningful inclusion is possible when professionals come together as champions of learning and listeners of students' voices.

Chandra

INTERDEPENDENCE AND INCLUSION

The more I immerse myself in the narratives of speaking, minimally speaking, and non-speaking autistic people, the more aware I have become of how profoundly mistreated autistic people are in education and society and the ensuing effects on their school achievement and states of well-being. While I hesitate to share this thought because it is noticeably ableist, it deserves attention because it indicates that the autistic community's massive efforts to reclaim their voices are working. Personally and professionally, I am much more aware of loud, token, and missing voices and how particular narratives are used to defend positions of power. I am also more aware of how knowledge construction is influenced by both what is said and left unsaid. Researchers and educators need to strengthen our listening practices to ensure diverse and even opposing voices are equally considered in ideas and decisions on what it means for students to be authentically included in education. Ethical listening practices, including the opportunity for self-representation of non and minimally speaking voices, help to re-balance power dynamics that have led to the pathologizing of autism and disability and the overuse of strategies that aim to remediate. Researchers, educators, and autism allies also need to find ways to mainstream inclusive practices to relieve the massive pressure on the autistic community to "solve problems [and injustices] they did not create" (Kapp, 2020, p.10). As Sinclair (1993) states, "We need you. We need your help and your understanding. Your world is not very open to us, and we would not make it without your strong support" (para.17).

This leads me to the recent global reality, the COVID-19 pandemic. In response to people's unfamiliar feelings of loneliness, isolation, and fear during the pandemic, autistic Maxfield Sparrow addressed autistic comrades in their blog post titled "Autistic in the Pandemic: A Call to Action" (March 19, 2020). Sparrow encouraged autistic people to resist the temptation to jest about non-autistics having to social distance, self-isolate, and feel the impacts of social exclusion. Instead, Sparrow stated with pride that "it's time to own [that we have spent our entire lives preparing for social distancing] and talk about our possible roles in this historical time" (para. 2). Sparrow goes on to say:

> *Be patient with them – coping with being alone is a skill like any other. We have had more chances to practice it, just as people with majority neurotypes have had more opportunities than us to practice socialization. Now we are the experts, and they are the ones who are deficient in a needed skill. We can help them, and we can do it with*

Chapter 7: Final Reflections

> *more kindness and compassion than many of us experienced at the hands of "helping" professionals in the past. So many of us are experts at loving without touching.*

Although Sparrow's recommendations concern a global health crisis, his compassionate response towards a society that repeatedly offers misunderstanding and mistreatment is timeless because it emphasizes the value of diversity in building and maintaining strong interdependent communities—a necessary characteristic of inclusive schools.

REFERENCES

Ahmed, S. (2002). This other and other others. *Economy and Society, 31*(4), 558-572.

Ashby, C., & Causton-Theoharis, J. (2009). Disqualified by the human race: A close reading of the autobiographies of individuals identified as autistic. *International Journal of Inclusive Education, 13*(5), 501–516. https://doi.org/10.1080/13603110801886673

Attwood, T. (1997). Asperger's syndrome: A guide for parents and professionals. Jessica Kinsley Publishers.

Barnes, C., & Oliver, M. (2012). The New Politics of Disablement. Palgrave Macmillian, Eastbourne.

Bascom, J. (2012). Quiet hands. In J. Bascom (Ed.), *Loud hands:* Autistic People, Speaking (pp. 177–183). The Autistic Press.

Bergenmar, J., Rosqvist, H. B., & Lönngren, A. S. (2015). Autism and the question of the human. *Literature and Medicine, 33*(1), 202–221. https://doi.org/10.1353/lm.2015.0009

Bettleheim, B. (1967). The empty fortress: Infantile Autism and the birth of the self. The Free Press.

Beukelman, D., & Mirenda, P. (2005). Augmentative & alternative communication: Supporting children & adults with complex communication needs (3rd ed.). Paul H. Brookes.

Brookfield, S. D. (2017). *Becoming a critically reflective teacher* (2nd ed.). Jossey-Bass.

Brown, L. (2011). The significance of semantics: Person first language: Why it matters. Autistic Hoya. https://autistichoya.com/2011/08/significance-of-semantics-person-first.html

Cage, E., Di Monaco, J., & Newell, V. (2018). Experiences of autism acceptance and mental health in autistic adults. *Journal of Autism and Developmental Disorders, 48*, 473–484. https://doi.org/10.1007/s10803-017-3342-7

Chamak, B. (2008). Autism and social movements: French parents' associations and international autistic individuals' organisations. *Sociology of Health & Illness, 30*(1), 76–96. https://doi.org/10.1111/j.1467-9566.2007.01053.x

Chandrasekhar, T., & Sikich, L. (2015). Challenges in the diagnosis and treatment of depression in autism spectrum disorders across the lifespan. *Dialogues in Clinical Neuroscience, 17*(2), 219–227. https://doi.org/10.31887/DCNS.2015.17.2/tchandrasekhar

Chown, N., Robinson, J., Beardon, L., Dwoning, J. Hughes, L. Leatherland, J., fox, K., Hickman, L., & MacGregor, D., (2017). Improving research about us, with us: A draft framework for inclusive autism research. Disability & Society, 32(5), 720-734. https://doi.org/10.1080/09687599.2017.1320273

Convention on the rights of the child (1989) Treaty no. 27531. *United Nations Treaty Series*, 1577, pp. 3-178.

Danker, J., Strnadova, I., & Cumming, T. (2016). School experiences of students with autism spectrum disorder within the context of student wellbeing: A review and analysis of the literature. *Australasian Journal of Special Education, 40*(1), 59–78. https://doi.org/10.1017/jse.2016.1

Denzin, N. K. (1989). *Interpretive biography.* Sage Publications, Inc.

DePape, A.-M., & Lindsay, S. (2016). Lived experiences from the perspective of individuals with autism spectrum disorder: A qualitative meta-synthesis. *Focus on Autism and Other Developmental Disabilities, 31*(1), 60–71. https://doi.org/10.1177/1088357615587504

Dillon, G., Underwood, J., & Freemantle, L. (2016). Autism and the U.K. secondary school experience. *Focus on Autism and Other Developmental Disabilities, 31*(3), 221–230. https://doi.org/10.1177/1088357614539833

Dolezal, L. (2017). Representing posthuman embodiment: Considering feasibility and the case of Aimee Mullins. *Women's Studies, 46*(1), 60–75. https://doi.org/10.1080/00497878.2017.1252569

Domović, V., Vidović Vlasta, V., & Bouillet, V. (2017). Student teachers' beliefs about the teachers' role in inclusive education. *European Journal of Special Needs Education, 32*(2), 175–190. https://doi.org/10.1080/08856257.2016.1194571

Donvan, J., & Zucker, C. (2016). In a different key: The story of Autism. Broadway Books.

Eisenberg, L. & Kanner, L. (1956). Childhood schizophrenia: Symposium, 1955:6. Early infantile autism, 1943-1955. *The American Journal of Orthopsychiatry, 26*(3), 556–566. https://doi.org/10.1111/j.1939-0025.1956.tb06202.x

Ellsworth, E. (1997). Teaching positions: Difference, pedagogy, and the Power of Address. New Teachers College Press.

Fernell, E., Giacobini, M., Gillberg, C., Lundstrom, S., Olsson, M., & Westerlund, J. (2015). "Recovery" from the diagnosis of autism -and Then? *Neuropsychiatric Disease and Treatment, 7*(11), 999–1005.

French, D. P., & Hankins, M. (2003). The expectancy-value muddle in the theory of planned behaviour--and some proposed solutions. *British Journal of Health Psychology, 8*(1), 37–55. https://doi.org/10.1348/135910703762879192

Frith, U. (1991). Autistic psychopathy in childhood. *In Autism and Asperger Syndrome* (pp. 37–92). https://doi.org/10.1017/CBO9780511526770.002

Ganz, J. (2014). Aided augmentative and alternative communication for people with ASD. Springer.

Global Education Monitoring Report. (2020). *Global education monitoring report, 2020: Inclusion and education: All means all – UNESCO Digital Library*.UNESCO. https://unesdoc.unesco.org/ark://48223/pf0000373718

Goodley, D., Lawthom, R., & Runswick-Cole, K. (2014). Posthuman disability studies. *Subjectivity, 7*, 342–361. https://doi.org/10.1057/sub.2014.15

Goodley, D., & Runswick-Cole, K. (2016). Becoming dishuman: Thinking about the human through dis/ability. *Discourse (Berkeley, Calif.), 37*(1), 1–15. https://doi.org/10.1080/01596306.2014.930021

Graham, L.J. (2020) *Inclusive education in the 21st century*. In Graham, L.J. (Ed.) Inclusive Education for the 21st Century: Theory, Policy and Practice, (pp. 3–26). Routledge.

Graham, L.J., Medhurst, M., Tancredi, H., Spandagou, I., Walton, E. (2020) *Fundamental concepts of inclusive education*. In Graham, L.J. (Ed.) Inclusive Education for the 21st Century: Theory, Policy and Practice, (pp. 27–54). Routledge.

Graveline, F.J. (1998). *First voice as critical pedagogy*. Circle works: Transforming Eurocentric consciousness. Fernwood.

Greydanus, D., & Toledo-Pereyra, L. (2012). Historical perspectives on autism: It's record of discovery and its present state of slipsism, skepticism, and sorrowful suspicion. *Pediatric Clinics of North America, 59*(1), 1–11. https://doi.org/10.1016/j.pcl.2011.10.004

Gruson-Wood, J.F. (2016). Autism, expert discourses, and subjectification: A critical examination of applied behavioural therapies. *Studies in Social Justice, 10*(1), 38–58. https://doi.org/10.26522/ssj.v10i1.1331

Haug, P. (2017). Understanding inclusive education: Ideals and reality. *Scandinavian Journal of Disability Research, 19*(3), 206–217. https://doi.org/10.1080/15017419.2016.1224778

Higashida, N. (2016). The reason I jump: The inner voice of a thirteen-year-old boy with Autism. Random House Trade Paperbacks.

Hippler, K., & Klicpera, C. (2003). A retrospective analysis of the clinical case records of 'autistic psychopaths' diagnosed by Hans Asperger and his team at the University Children's Hospital Vienna. *Philosophical Transactions of the Royal Society of London. Series B, Biological Sciences, 358*(1430), 291–301. https://doi.org/10.1098/rstb.2002.1197

Humphrey, N., & Lewis, S. (2008). What does "inclusion" mean for pupils on the autistic spectrum in mainstream secondary schools? *Journal of Research in Special Educational Needs, 8*(3), 132–140. https://doi.org/10.1111/j.1471-3802.2008.00115.x

International Society for Augmentative and Alternative Communication. (2014). ISAAC position statement on Facilitated Communication. *Augmentative and Alternative Communication, 4*(30), 357–358. https://doi.org/10.3109/07434618.2014.971492

Jaswal, V.K., Wayne, A. & Golino, H. (2020). Eye-tracking reveals agency in assisted autistic communication. SciRep, 10, 7882. https://doi.org/10.1038/s41598-020-64553-9

Kasari, C., Kaiser, A., Goods, K., Nietfeld, J., Mathy, P., Landa, R., Murphy, S., & Almirall, D. (2014). Communication interventions for minimally verbal children with autism: A sequential multiple assignment randomized trial. *Journal of the American Academy of Child and Adolescent Psychiatry, 53*(6), 635–646. https://doi.org/10.1016/j.jaac.2014.01.019

Kedar, I. (2018, October 5). The 3 p's of communication skeptics. *Ido in Autismland*. http://idoinautismland.com/?p=779

Kenny, L., Hattersley, C., Molins, B., Buckley, C., Povey, C., & Pellicano, E. (2015). Which terms should be used to describe autism? Perspectives from the UK autism community. *Autism, 20*(4), 442–462. https://doi.org/10.1177/1362361315588200

Kirkham, P. (2017). 'The line between intervention and abuse'– autism and applied behaviour analysis. *History of the Human Sciences, 30*, 107–126. Advanced online publication. https://doi.org/10.1177/0952695117702571

Kotsopoulos, S. (2014). The parents of the child with autism. *Encephalos, 51*(1943), 23–27.

Kumashiro, K. (2002). Against repetition: Addressing resistance to anti-oppressive change in the practices of learning, teaching, supervising, and researching. *Harvard Educational Review, 72*(1), 67–93. https://doi.org/10.17763/haer.72.1.c11617526l7k46v6

Lebenhagen, C. (2022). Autistic Students' Views on Meaningful Inclusion: A Canadian Perspective. *Journal of Education. 1-16* https://doi.org/10.1177/00220574221101378

Lebenhagen, C. (2019). Including speaking and non-speaking voice in research. *Autism in Adulthood*, 2, 128-131. https://doi.org/10.1089/aut.2019.0002

Lovaas, O. I., & Buch, G. (1997). Intensive behavioral intervention with young children with autism. In N. N. Singh (Ed.), Prevention and treatment of severe behavior problems: Models and methods in developmental disabilities (pp. 61–86). Thomson Brooks/Cole Publishing Co.

Moen, T. (2006). Reflections on the Narrative Research Approach. *International Journal of Qualitative Methods*, 56–69. https://doi.org/10.1177/160940690600500405

McNiff, J. (2013). Action research (3rd ed.). Routledge.

McCrimmon, A. (2015). Inclusive Education in Canada. [SAGE Publications Ltd.]. *Intervention in School and Clinic, 50*(4), 234–237. https://doi.org/10.1177/1053451214546402

Merriam-Webster. (n.d.). Aut-. In *Merriam-Webster.com dictionary*. https://www.merriam-webster.com/dictionary/aut-

Messiou, K. (2019). The missing voices: Students as a catalyst for promoting inclusive education. *International Journal of Inclusive Education, 23*(7-8), 768–781.

https://doi.org/10.1080/13603116.2019.1623326

Milton, D. (2016) Re-thinking autism: diagnosis, identity and equality, *Disability & Society, 31*(10), 1413-1415. DOI: 10.1080/09687599.2016.1221666

Mitchell, D. (2017). Almost everything I'd been told about my son's autism was wrong. *New Statesman America*. https://www.newstatesman.com/culture/books/2017/07/david-mitchell-almost-everything-i-d-been-told-about-my-son-s-autism-was-wrong

MTOWN97. (2019, April 17). Violent ableism: A Structural Epidemic. UAB Institute for Human Rights Blog. https://sites.uab.edu/humanrights/author/mtown97/

National Institute of Drug Abuse. (January, 2016). *What are hallucinogens?* https://web.archive.org/web/20160417180046/https:/wwwdrugabuse.gov/publications/drugfacts/hallucinogens

Neumärker, K. (2003). Leo Kanner: His years in Berlin, 1906 – 24. The roots of autistic disorder. *History of Psychiatry, 14*(2), 205–218. https://doi.org/10.1177/0957154X030142005

Ospina, M., Krebs-Seida, J., Clark, B., Karkhaneh, M., Hartling, L., Tjosvold, L., Vandermeer, B., & Smith, V. (2008). Behavioural and developmental interventions for autism spectrum disorder: A clinical systematic review. *PLoS One, 3*, e3755. Advance online publication. https://doi.org/10.1371/journal.pone.0003755

Pitt, A., & Britzman, D. (2003). Speculations on qualities of difficult knowledge in teaching and learning: An experiment in psychoanalytic research. *International Journal of Qualitative Studies in Education: QSE, 16*(6), 755–776. https://doi.org/10.1080/09518390310001632135

Pollack, R. (1997). *The Creation of Dr. B: A Biography of Bruno Bettelheim by Richard. Pollak.* Simon. & Schuster.

Reis, S.M., Gelbar, N.W. & Madaus, J.W. (2021). Understanding the Academic Success of Academically Talented College Students with Autism Spectrum Disorders. *J Autism Dev Disord*. https://doi.org/10.1007/s10803-021-05290-4

Roberts, J., & Webster, A. (2020). Including students with autism in schools: a whole school approach to improve outcomes for students with autism. *International Journal of inclusive Education*. https://www.tandfonline.com/doi/full/10.1080/13603116.2020.1712622 https://doi.org/10.1080/13603116.2020.1712622

Saggers, B. (2015). Student perceptions: Improving the educational experiences of high school students on the autism spectrum. *Improving Schools, 18*(1), 35–45. https://doi.org/10.1177/1365480214566213

Sallows, G., & Graupner, T. (2005). Intensive behavioral treatment for children with autism: Four-year outcome and predictors. *American Journal of Mental Retardation, 110*(6), 417–438. https://doi.org/10.1352/0895-8017(2005)110[417:IBTFCW]2.0.CO;2

Saloviita, T., Leppänen, M., & Ojalammi, U. (2014). Authorship in facilitated communication: An analysis of 11 cases. *Augmentative and Alternative Communication, 30*, 213-225.

Saur, E., & Sidorkin, A. (2018). Disability, dialogue, and the posthuman. *Studies in Philosophy and Education, 37*, 567–568. https://doi.org/10.1007/s11217-018-9616-5

St. Pierre, J. (2015). Cripping communication: Speech, disability, and exclusion in liberal humanist and posthumanist discourse. *Communication Theory, 25*(3), 330–348. https://doi.org/10.1111/comt.12054

Scheffer, E. (2018). Asperger's children: The origins of Autism in Nazi Vienna. Norton & Company.

Sigafoos, J., Green, V., Edrisinha, C., & Lancioni, G. (2007). Flashback to the 1960s: LSD in the treatment of autism. *Developmental Neurorehabilitation, 10*(1), 75–81. https://doi.org/10.1080/13638490601106277

Socially Anxious Advocate. (2015). *Why I left ABA.* https://sociallyanxiousadvocate.wordpress.com/2015/05/22/why-i-left-aba/ Stuart, M. (2016). Routledge.

Sparrow, M. (2020, March 19). Autistic in the pandemic: A call to action. *Thinking Person's Guide to Autism.* http://www.thinkingautismguide.com/2020/03/autistic-in-pandemic-call-to-action.htm

Stop Ableism. (2019). *What is ableism?* http://www.stopableism.org/p/what-is-ableism.html

Sullivan, G. M., & Artino, A. R., Jr. (2013). Analyzing and interpreting data From Likert-Type Scales. *Journal of Graduate Medical Education, 5*(4), 541–542. https://doi.org/10.4300/JGME-5-4-18

Tager-Flusberg, H., & Kasari, C. (2013, December). Minimally verbal school-aged children with autism spectrum disorder: The neglected end of the spectrum. *Autism Research, 6,* 468–478. Advance online publication. https://doi.org/10.1002/aur.1329

Tangen, R. (2005). Promoting inclusive education in secondary school in Norway: A national programme for teacher development. *European Journal of Special Needs Education, 20*(1), 57–70. https://doi.org/10.1080/0885625042000319089

Taylor, C. (1992). The politics of recognition. In C. Taylor & A. Gutmann (Eds.), Multi-Culturalism and 'The Politics of Recognition. Princeton University Press.

Thompson, S. A., Lyons, W., & Timmons, V. (2015). Inclusive education policy: What the leadership of Canadian teacher associations has to say about it. *International Journal of Inclusive Education, 19*(2), 121–140. https://doi.org/10.1080/13603116.2014.908964

Time Magazine. (1948). *Medicine: Frosted children.*

http://autismedsp5310s20f10.pbworks.com/f/Time-Medicine_+Frosted+Children+--+Printout.pdf

Tisdall, E. (2012). The challenge and challenging of childhood studies? Learning from disability studies and research with disabled children. *Children & Society, 26*(3), 181–191. https://doi.org/10.1111/j.1099-0860.2012.00431.x

Todd, S. (2003). Listening as an attentiveness to 'dense plots. In Learning from the Other: Levinas, Psychoanalysis, and Ethical Possibilities in Education (pp. 117–140). SUNY Press.

Towle, H. (2015). *Disability and inclusion in Canadian education: Policy, procedure, and practice*. Canadian Centre for Policy Alternatives. National Office.

UNESCO. (1994). *The Salamanca Statement and Framework for Action on Special Needs Education*. Adopted by the World Conference on Special Needs Education: Access and Quality. Salamanca, Spain, 7-10 June. U.

United Nations. (1989). Convention on the rights of the child, office of the high commissioner. United Nations.

United Nations. (2006). *Convention on the rights of persons with disabilities*. http://www.refworld.org/docid/4680cd212.html

Vanerheiden, G. (2002). A journey through early augmentative communication and computer access. *Journal of Rehabilitation Research and Development, 39*(6), 39–53.

Verhoeff, B. (2013). Autism in flux: A history of the concept from Leo Kanner to DSM-5. *History of Psychiatry, 24*(4), 442–458. https://doi.org/10.1177/0957154X13500584

Waltz, M. (2005). Reading case studies of people with autistic spectrum disorders: A cultural studies approach to issues of disability representation. *Disability & Society, 20*, 421–435. Advance online publication. https://doi.org/10.1080/09687590500086575

Weiss, J., & Delmolino, L. (2006). The relationship between early learning rates and treatment outcome for children with autism receiving intensive home-based applied behaviour analysis. *The Behavior Analyst Today, 7*(1), 96–110. https://doi.org/10.1037/h0100140

Woodfield, C., & Ashby, C. (2016). "The right path of equality": Supporting high school students with autism who type to communicate. *International Journal of Inclusive Education, 20*(4), 435–454. https://doi.org/10.1080/13603116.2015.1088581

Wurtzburg, S., & Campbell, L. (1995). North American Indian sign language: Evidence of its existence before European contact. *International Journal of American Linguistics, 61*(2), 153–167. https://doi.org/10.1086/466249

Wing, L. (1981). Asperger's syndrome: A clinical account. *Psychological Medicine, 11*(1), 115–129. https://doi.org/10.1017/S0033291700053332

Wood, A. (2016). Temple Grandin: Voice for the voiceless. Skyhorse Publishing.

Zager, D., Wehmeyer, M., & Simpson, R. (2012). Educating students with autism spectrum disorders: Research-based principles and practices. *Intervention in School and Clinic, 50*(4), 234–237.

Zeldovich, L. (2018). How history forgot the women who defined autism. *Spectrum: Autism Research News*. https://www.spectrumnews.org/features/deep-dive/history-forgot-woman-defined-autism/

Zeliadt, N. (2018). Revealing autism's hidden strengths. *SpectrumNews*. https://www.spectrumnews.org/features/deep-dive/revealing-autisms-hidden-strengths/

ABOUT THE AUTHORS

Anantha Krishnamurthy is a minimally speaking autistic teen. He is an avid Math enthusiast passionate about pursuing a STEM (Science, Technology, Engineering, and Math) education. When Anantha is not dreaming about STEM, he has grand designs of becoming a fiery writer, shooting down barriers autistic people face with his words. Anantha regularly publishes his poetry on Neuroclastic and his blog, Anantha Muses (anantha-muses.blogspot.com). Anantha has constant cravings for friendships and donuts.

Janani Ramanath is trained as an architect, has a master's degree in architectural lighting design, and works as a freelance lighting designer in Calgary, Alberta. Her parenting journey has taken her through many unexpected albeit interesting twists and turns. She is passionate about communication rights, presuming competence and inclusive education. Unwinding with novels or movies is her guilty pleasure.

Robert Choate is an educator that specializes in inclusive best practices for autistic students. He has worked with neurodivergent youth for his entire career and strives to be a strong advocate and ally for those voices that are not always heard. He is excited about the growing momentum to do right by and learn from diverse learners. Robert enjoys spending time in nature with his dog Harley in his free time.

Chandra Lebenhagen has been an educator and autism ally for over 20 years. She recently completed a doctoral degree in curriculum and education, where her research explored the self-reported school experiences of autistic youth in Canada. Through her private practice and various research and writing projects, Chandra aims to work with others to help dismantle and reshape ableist systems and methods in research and education. She never tires of coffee and the Rocky Mountains.

CPSIA information can be obtained
at www.ICGtesting.com
Printed in the USA
BVHW070727111122
651210BV00001B/2

9 781039 154049